The Infantile in Psychoanalytic Practice Today

The Infantile in Psychoanalytic Practice Today demonstrates the concept of the Infantile, first proposed almost a quarter of a century ago, and the ways in which it has become an indispensable tool in contemporary psychoanalytic clinical practice.

As a "concept of the third type", the Infantile makes the "links-between-the-links" woven into the transference/countertransference functional and effective with patients of all ages, and is related to the double helix between infant neurosis and transference neurosis as revealed by Freud. The author proposes the Infantile as a key concept in the psychic organization of every human being, as the unconscious internal space that includes both the repressed elements of the past and the constantly renewed expressions of the drives. As a unique and dynamic configuration for each person, the book explores the way this relates to others, to the environment, and also to the individual's own psychic contents and movements.

This eagerly awaited English edition includes two new chapters, filling a gap in the psychoanalytic library. As a concept with international scope, these writings on the Infantile will be essential reading for psychoanalysts working today and all those interested in the history of psychoanalysis.

Florence Guignard is a Franco-Swiss psychoanalyst and honorary full member of the Paris Psychoanalytical Society (SPP), as well as a training member in child and adolescent psychoanalysis of the International Psychoanalytical Association. She is the author of numerous books, including *Psychoanalytic Concepts and Technique in Development: Psychoanalysis, Neuroscience and Physics* (Routledge).

Psychoanalytic Ideas and Applications Series

IPA Publications Committee

Recent titles in the Series include

Permanent Disquiet
Psychoanalysis and the Transitional Subject
Michel de M'Uzan

Psychoanalytic Work with Families and Couples
Clinical Perspectives on Suffering
Susana Kuras Mauer, Sara Moscona, and Silvia Resnizky

Narcissistic Fantasies in Film and Fiction
Masters of the Universe
Ilany Kogan

Psychoanalytic Reflections on Writing, Cinema and the Arts
Facing Beauty and Loss
Paola Golinelli

Change Through Time in Psychoanalysis
Transformations and Interventions, The Three Level Model
Margaret Ann Fitzpatrick Hanly, Marina Altmann de Litvan, Ricardo Bernardi

The Infantile in Psychoanalytic Practice Today
Florence Guignard

The Infantile in Psychoanalytic Practice Today

Florence Guignard

Translated by Andrew Weller

Routledge
Taylor & Francis Group
LONDON AND NEW YORK

First published 2022
by Routledge
2 Park Square, Milton Park, Abingdon, Oxon OX14 4RN

and by Routledge
605 Third Avenue, New York, NY 10158

Routledge is an imprint of the Taylor & Francis Group, an informa business

British Library Cataloguing-in-Publication Data
A catalogue record for this book is available from the British Library

Library of Congress Cataloging-in-Publication Data
Names: Guignard, Florence, author.
Title: The infantile in psychoanalytic practice today / Florence Guignard ; translated by Andrew Weller.
Other titles: Au vif de l'infantile. English
Description: Abingdon, Oxon ; New York, NY : Routledge, 2022. | Series: The international psychoanalytical association psychoanalytic ideas and applications series | Includes bibliographical references and index.
Identifiers: LCCN 2021008545 (print) | LCCN 2021008546 (ebook) | ISBN 9781032049779 (hardback) | ISBN 9781032049755 (paperback) | ISBN 9781003195436 (ebook)
Subjects: LCSH: Infant psychology. | Infant analysis. | Sex (Psychology) | Psychoanalysis.
Classification: LCC BF719 .G8413 2022 (print) | LCC BF719 (ebook) | DDC 155.42/2—dc23
LC record available at https://lccn.loc.gov/2021008545
LC ebook record available at https://lccn.loc.gov/2021008546

ISBN: 978-1-032-04977-9 (hbk)
ISBN: 978-1-032-04975-5 (pbk)
ISBN: 978-1-003-19543-6 (ebk)

Typeset in Times New Roman
by Apex CoVantage, LLC

"A psychic place of primary and unrepresentable drive emergences on the boundary of the *Ucs.* and the *Pcs.*, the Infantile is the most acute point of our affects, the locus of hope and cruelty, of courage and unconcern; it operates throughout life, in a twin spiral of process and assignment of meaning. . . . In its metaphorical aspect, the concept also applies to its hallucinatory and proto-symbolic retinue of preforms that are constantly evolving in all our mental activities". Florence Guignard (*The Infantile in Psychoanalytic Practice Today,* p. xx)

Contents

French editor's note

In 1996, Florence Guignard published *Au vif de l'infantile: réflexions sur la situation analytique* Guignard, 1996). Although it was her first book, the author was no longer in the early stages of her intellectual journey since she had already developed original and rigorous lines of thought in around one hundred scientific articles and contributions to collective works, and also through her participation in numerous seminars, congresses and international conferences. Florence Guignard chose to sew this book, which collates ten years of reflections and theoretical-clinical exchanges, with the *bright* red thread of the Infantile. This conceptual "selected fact" of course owed nothing to chance, for recognition of the child's speech, albeit concealed within the discourse of the adult, was already at the centre of the author's concerns. In her words, this concept still had, however, "to acquire its capital letter and its credentials", that is to say, perhaps, it had to break the glass ceiling of child psychoanalysis that some "serious" psychoanalysts hastened to place above her head – it is worth recalling that Florence Guignard founded with Annie Anzieu, who sadly died during the preparation of this book, the Association of Child Psychoanalysis (APE), then the European Society for Child and Adolescent Psychoanalysis (SEPEA) – and to establish itself as a transversal psychoanalytic concept, animating infants as well as the elderly.

The concept of the Infantile took up this challenge, in France and around the world, winning the enthusiasm of its readership on each occasion. The success of the book in France and in French-speaking countries resulted in its reissue in 2002, but the unfortunate closure of the collection "Champs psychanalytiques" (Delachaux & Niestlé) left the book out of print, unlike the concept, which, itself, boldly continued its journey through the clinical field of the third millennium. Anxious to fill such an editorial gap in contemporary psychoanalysis, Ithaque offers this new edition reviewed by the author, embellished with an updating of the bibliography and enlarged by two new chapters and an index.

Florence Guignard's long experience as a translator, as well as her polyglot culture, led her to carefully consider the question of French translations transcribed in *Au vif de l'Infantile, aujourd'hui*. This is why the French *"identification projective"* (an awkward translation, according to her, of "projective identification") here gives way to *"projection identificatoire"* in order to ensure the primacy, both syntactic and conceptual, of the projective dimension over the identificatory dimension. Likewise, it was a deliberate editorial choice to prefer the first French translations of the Freudian texts – or even, on occasion, translations of Florence Guignard from her personal reading of the German edition – rather than the *Œuvres complètes*, sometimes too literal and not always honouring the literary dispositions of Sigmund Freud. We would like to warmly thank Florence Guignard, who participated, with her characteristic energy, in the renewal of her *first* book, which over time has become a classic in psychoanalysis. The time it took to produce this new edition offered us a great opportunity to "sejourn in the limbo of children" (Pontalis, 1998, p. 11) and to become familiar, as much as possible at least, with the palpitations of the Infantile present in everyone, and even an editor.

Jérémy Tancray

Series editor's foreword

The Publications Committee of the International Psychoanalytic Association continues, with the present volume, the Psychoanalytic Ideas and Applications series.

The aim of this series is to focus on the scientific production of significant authors whose works are outstanding contributions to the development of the psychoanalytic field and to set out relevant ideas and themes, generated during the history of psychoanalysis, that deserve to be known and discussed by present day psychoanalysts.

The relationship between psychoanalytic ideas and their applications needs to be put forward from the perspective of theory, clinical practice and research, in order to maintain their validity for contemporary psychoanalysis.

The Publication's Committee's objective is to share these ideas with the psychoanalytic community and with professionals in other related disciplines so as to expand their knowledge and generate a productive interchange between the text and the reader. The IPA Publications Committee is pleased to publish the revised English version of the book *The Infantile in Psychoanalytic Practice Today* by Florence Guignard which was first published in French in 1996.

In this book, Guignard gathers her theoretical and clinical views of the last ten years. She does so by following the common thread of the notion of the Infantile. In doing so, she masterfully takes us through a most interesting journey that conveys the many theoretical and clinical facets of this essential psychoanalytic notion which has become central in psychoanalytic thinking.

Guignard arrives at a most original and rich definition of the Infantile:

> The infantile is a basic structure on the fringes of our animal nature, the depository and container of our drives, be they libidinal or hateful on the one hand or epistemophilic on the other. It is that combination of drive-related and flexible structural elements that makes a person who he is and not someone else. Irreducible, unique and hence

> universal, the infantile is therefore the entity that will usher in our mental life, through all the developments of its psychic bisexuality as organized by the Oedipus complex.
>
> (p. 16)

Throughout the book one can recognise and appreciate her concern for the historic development of psychoanalytic theory and its future as well as the rigour of her continuous search to articulate concepts from different psychoanalytic cultures. Her knowledge and mastery of psychoanalysts from different regions of the world is remarkable.

Skilfully organized in sixteen chapters, the book covers a myriad of perspectives: from Freud's notion of the Infantile, child and adolescent psychoanalysis to female auto-erotism. Clinical considerations run all through the book.

There is little doubt that this book is a remarkable contribution to the topic of the Infantile. One should be thankful to Dr. Guignard for her insightful and creative contribution. At the end of her book, the author wonders whether the reader will find that "the heart of the Infantile has run tight through the pages of her book" (p. 179). There is no doubt that the author has been greatly successful in her endeavour.

Gabriela Legorreta
Series Editor
Chair, IPA Publications Committee

Preface

This volume is devoted to the little *child of yesteryear*, living forever at another level of psychic functioning and in another temporality, and caught up in the incessant work of the evolving unconscious – work that is functional for its growth, its potential of existence, and its self. This *child of yesteryear*, who is the subjective archivist of anxieties, splits and repressions but also of the imprints left by his family (maternal, paternal, fraternal), remains forever the subjective judge of the way in which his needs and desires were taken into account. As a subject of the unconscious, he assumes an ineffable character due to the historical/ahistorical condition which is his own. As an object of analytical work, he is constituted there as a third presence (Ogden, 2004), a kind of fantasized *alter ego* in the session, an imaginary brother created/found where the historical memory of early childhood is brought to mind much less often than that of the senses and affects, *memories in feelings* (Klein, 1957).

With the clarity that characterizes her conceptualizations, Florence Guignard leads us here as closely as possible towards this "Infantile", more exactly as closely as possible towards the aspects and points of impact that it assumes in the session, both for the patient and analyst alike. Albeit a fleeting phenomenon owing to its somewhat "polymorphously perverse" appearance (Freud, 1905), this Infantile may be conceived as a figure identified and created by the "analysing situation" (Donnet, 2005), as much as a "co-thinking" (Widlöcher, 2013) of two minds at work confronted with symbolization which has not yet materialized. These two minds observe themselves functioning and listen to each other being listened to under the regressive potential effect of a clinical method that organizes an analytical space (Viderman, 1970) or analytical field (Baranger & Baranger, 1961–62) that is capable of *containing and transforming* the derivatives of unconscious communications.

If the concept of "infantile sexuality", along with its neurosis, is just as central as that of "transference" and "unconscious" in psychoanalysis, its theorizations are called upon to evolve for the benefit of listening and interpretability during the session. Unlike postulates, any theoretical definition of concepts and notions leads to the search for a better fit between the theoretical-technical tools and the characteristics of the object studied. In psychoanalysis, as in any discipline, there is an interest in distinguishing the status of discoveries from that of theorizations about them. Discoveries remain, theories evolve. . .

This is what clearly motivates the project of Florence Guignard's book. In her attempt to delimit the concept of the Infantile again, the author wishes to articulate concepts derived from Freudian and post-Freudian psychoanalytic models, models that have gradually established themselves as extensions of metapsychology. Melanie Klein, Wilfred Bion, Donald Meltzer, and sometimes Donald Winnicott, are the authors Florence Guignard refers to most; they each contributed in an original way to founding bipersonal models of the psyche and, mutatis mutandis, of the analytical situation. The inexhaustible questions of the "how" and the "why" of suffering in psychic life, led them to give only a descriptive value – unipersonal – to the Freudian drive model.

Such an evolution requires the most important clarifications when using concepts. In this book, the "required" exercise is significant because Florence Guignard contrasts the concept of Infantile with the notion of infantile, more general in child psychoanalysis, used sometimes to describe the experience of a subjective state, sometimes as part of a nominal phrase for a structured organization, as in "infantile neurosis". Before letting the reader discover the angles of approach to the Infantile chosen by the author – all of which are possible vertexes – and appreciate her theoretical propositions, I do not think it superfluous to place them within a contemporary psychoanalytic line of thought, since the perspectives she offers provide the tools to tackle the essential subject of the Infantile in psychoanalysis. Freudian metapsychology is indeed the point of origin and anchor of the cognitive adventure relating to the "new object" defined, namely, the dynamic unconscious. However, over the different generations of analysts and the expansion of clinical experience, we have witnessed the emergence of a new generation of concepts giving rise to the formulation of new theoretical-clinical models, whose compliance with Freudian indications is variable, bringing to the table of psychoanalysts the question of the practice of "commensality", as Florence Guignard evokes in this book.

Could it be otherwise? Although the tree of analytical knowledge has its roots in the vast and complex Freudian corpus, it is nonetheless presented as an "open work" (Ferro, 1996) linked to the generativity proper to its method. The method can be envisaged as a sort of probe working to widen the passages, in constant formation, between the unconscious and the conscious, between the body-ego and the thinking-ego (Anzieu, 1994) giving rise to a growth in the possibilities of thinking and dreaming, as well as of learning from and forgetting experiences. On another level, such potentiality will be reflected in theory and its descriptive models. Faced with its object, an unconscious that imposes itself and simultaneously conceals itself, theorizations can only proceed by approximation.

It was in fits and starts that a slow revision and enlargement was carried out compared to the initial centrality accorded to the instinctual drive model and to infantile psychosexuality, a model reconstructed on the basis of "transference neurosis". This slow and silent revision which, from a structural perspective, is anchored to a relational bipersonal perspective, played its part in the need to articulate the vicissitudes of drive accomplishments with the role provided by the object as a revealer and operator of the entanglement of drive impulses and their powerful expressions in phantasy, active from early times. The primary object/environment – perceived as part/whole (Klein, 1946; Fairbairn, 1952) – changes the intensity of the drive drama in the relationship. The phantasized relationships that the ego maintains with the maternal body, and with the paternal element that she carries within her, turn out to constitute a space-time of the passions, of *suffering*. They come from painful perceptions of bodily states specific to the self of the small child, projected/evacuated (magically) into the object by means of projective identification, a major mechanism on which Florence Guignard lingers in a fine chapter of this volume. This state of defensive fusion, primary and narcissistic, is deposed, under the effect of denials in reality, by other defensive manoeuvres: splitting, idealization of a part/good/bad quality of the object, with, as a bonus, attempts to repair this subjective-object so that it becomes another. The Infantile is thus somewhat redrawn in relation to the libidinal model of the stages described by Freud (1905) and Abraham (1924), since primary anxieties and Oedipal elements are postulated (Klein, 1932) as being active at a very early stage in the newborn. Part-object relations with oral and anal qualities, in danger of being quickly genitalized even before the onset of the phallic stage, lead Florence Guignard to underline the role of phantasy concerning the digestive tract in relation to the constitution of the primal scene.

This sexual dimension of the Infantile first acts as a guardian against massive dependence on the primary object (breast-penis), while waiting to reap the benefits of defusion and integration for the ego and its object, gleaned from the development of the *stations of the via crucis*: the development of the paranoid-schizoid and depressive positions (Klein, 1946), without forgetting, in the background, the autistic-contiguous position (Ogden, 1994). These psychic positions always remain active at certain levels and oscillate functionally according to the pain or trauma that the psyche has to deal with (Bion, 1962b), that is to say contents of experience that test the durability of the containers necessary for thought. It is thanks to introjections of the capacity to contain the offerings of psychic tools by the object/analyst, that the ego enters the zone of separability, that of a defusion without the risk of dissociative anxiety or melancholic loss. Access to the depressive position and to the work involved in coming to terms with the loss and renunciation of the object of infantile omnipotence with, as a reward, introjective identification with a good object – the equivalent at the level of thought of fertile copulation, leads persecutory anxieties to give way to castration anxieties which are more in line with the emergence of the Oedipal desires of the phallic-genital organization. Thanks to weaning and the onset of the depressive position, it is a psychic space with three protagonists that emerges. The diverse relationships and links between these protagonists lend themselves to the work of symbolization and unconscious phantasy (Segal, 1990) in the form of "infantile sexual theories". The latter therefore prove to be useful for "playing" with secondary identifications – with the maternal dimension (with its feminine element) and the paternal dimension (with its masculine element) – in order to organize the basic montage of bisexuality as gendered identity. It is therefore a question of living in a new, delimited and personal psychic space, where the shadow of the absent presence can be found and recreated in symbols, among which those of verbal language have great organizing power for thought.

While the Infantile of the initial stages of life, with its first forms of object-relations, works against the suffering linked to dependence and states of anxiety about death aroused in the process, its dramaturgy is placed under the sign of the need for "the helping object", where sexuation (or the gender aspect) of the relationship is only secondary. This is what sets it apart from the notion of desiring infantile sexuality, which is organized under the aegis of phallic-genital libido and castration anxiety, an agency of secondary repression with ideational connotations.

The *child of yesteryear*, who is forever evolving in the unconscious and, so to speak, "sustains himself" in the session with the help of the transference, brings just as much the Infantile in the infant – a "*vital/sexual*" (Laplanche) – driven by the need for a living libidinal helping object who counterbalances the great distress of the infant – as an "infantile/*sexual* driven by desire. The first takes the path of raw phantasy configurations, which are marked by greed and envy and exposed to the effects of the sadism of the superego and unconscious guilt. The phenomenon of "blind spots" in the analyst's countertransference work clearly shows the point of impact of the violence of this Infantile. Florence Guignard highlights the complexity of listening to material belonging to a level of violent and wild infantile organization, because it is less acceptable than that of a real infantile neurosis, whether it occurs in the child, adolescent or adult. If the infantile neurosis, in both the child and the adult, is already charged with a certain historicization of its desires and prohibitions, the Infantile of the pre-phallic period is marked more by the characteristics of implicit memory (Mancia, 2007). Their raw phantasies can then constitute a proto-symbolic state available for a work of "psychization", that is, a process of symbolization which will have to be accomplished within the analytical relationship, on the border of the id and the ego and on the frontiers of the unconscious and the conscious.

Florence Guignard thus reattributes value to the function of work specific to the preconscious, which she likens moreover to that provided by the "contact barrier" (Bion, 1962a): a territory par excellence for the fabrication of dream thought, a filter vis-à-vis "wild" instinctual drive activity just as much as brutal reality. The knowledge of the senses (perceptions, emotions, mental images) is here more than ever in the service of the evolving knowledge of the reflecting ego (linked ideas and secondary process thinking), which finds a mentor in the drive impulse K: knowledge, emotional truth.

Florence Guignard constantly emphasizes the equal worth that Bion grants to the drive impulse K compared to the other categories of impulses, grouped together as L (Love, life drive) and H (Hate, death drive), and even more to the importance of the positive and negative links that the K impulse maintains with each of these drive categories. These drive impulses, ranging from impersonal data to mode of functioning according to "group mentality" (Bion, 1962b), must, through transformation, achieve their personalizations in the solitude of the self in front of others. It is the same for the transition from a sexuality with a *narcissistic polarity*, that of infantile omnipotence, with the oral and anal possession of the mother/part object, to that of a *socialistic polarity* posterior to the depressive position, which "Oedipifies" the reality represented with a total and separate mother, restored to her husband, making it possible to *tolerate the uncertainty* of any encounter of otherness in the couple, family or group. This lack of certainty now becomes tolerable because it is contained within a framework of ensuring the safety of oneself and one's boundaries when faced with the range of one's own instinctual and representational heritage.

In her reading of the cases of Little Hans and young Leonardo, Florence Guignard highlights not only the creative destinies of the K impulse but also its obstacles, due to counter-truth (Gammil, 2007). Counter-truth is a poison of psychic life and of the analytic relationship, way of fleeing from the concern that needs to be shown for emotional truth (the Bionian "O").

It was not without arousing various resistances that the so-called "relational" analytical perspectives, identifiable in different ways in the works of Klein followed by Bion, Winnicott and their successors, began to be taken into consideration by French-speaking psychoanalysis. They accompanied the slow and silent revolution of psychoanalysis. These inflections and evolutions are to be considered in the first place for their influence on *the range of listening* in the session, but also on the "theorizing" work that precedes and accompanies the activity of interpretation – whether it be silent and/or formulated – until it concerns the practicability of benevolent "neutrality", of the interaction between the patient's "free associations" and the analyst's "evenly-suspended attention". This functional whole touches today on the very conception of the transference and countertransference as well as that of the function of bringing it under the aegis of what is known as "reverie" (Bion, 1962a; Grotstein, 2007; Ogden, 1997): that is what Florence Guignard's pages invite us to do.

Freud discovered transference in the context of a psychopathological situation, but he did not hesitate to recognize it as a general mechanism of psychic life. He also understood that it was an observable and interpretable mechanism, usable for treatment purposes. But what is transferred, ultimately? Above all, pain, excess mental suffering which seeks another object/subject with whom to share it. And in what forms and modalities does this appear during the session? More than other psychic states, these types of transference contents summon the presence of another (mind) which is receptive and thus supports the transformation of the subjective state of distress/suffering: the reference to the vicissitudes of the primary relationship is the prototype.

The transference is the product of an unconscious mechanism and conveys in itself the different levels of the psychic organization of the subject of the unconscious. These take on various forms in its action phantasies and in the degrees of symbolic and communicative shaping of its contents of experience. Such a characteristic means that, in the analysing situation, the transference(s), starting from the psychoneurosis and by means of the mechanism of reconstruction, must eventuate in an infantile neurosis capable of being converted into an analysable transference-neurosis. The transference neurosis is, however, in a constant oscillatory situation with the countertransference neurosis, making the analytical relationship the locus of the full edition of the transference, the total transference situation that Klein defended (Klein & Heimann, 1952).

Following the inflections and developments in psychoanalysis, we can recognize how much the transference in the session attracts not only the reactualization of the drive impulses, part or whole object relationships, and contrary or ambivalent feelings, but also preconceptions – innate or acquired – through this "something that has just been done by the subject", with its modality of perceiving and experiencing the object (Bion, 2005). In the transference, there are also proto-mental and pre-symbolic elements waiting to be born and to emerge at the heart of mental representations, of what is thinkable. This "something that has just been done by the subject" underlines the transformation that transference accomplishes through reverie. This is necessary in everyday life as in the analytic session. Transferring is just dreaming. It is only a question of effecting "dreamlike" transformations of perceptions and raw emotions in order to raise them to the domain of metaphor and meaning. The same goes for countertransference, with its introjective (Money-Kyrle, 1956) or projective (Grinberg, 2018) dispositions – an almost indissociable pair in the session, made up of crossed projective identifications and transprojective identifications (Feldman, 2009). They are only unconscious communications struggling to exorcise "demons" in the psyche: a past that does not pass, a promise of encounter and an anticipated new way of thinking.

This struggle is imposed on each of us in different ways on a daily basis, and crucially, it is true, in the analytic couple in session but also in groups, institutions and in the culture of the social domain.

Practising psychoanalysis with reasoned "faith" in this manner of proceeding and thinking about what is human involves watching over the state of activity of these demons and their evolution. This is what the author reminds us of in the last two chapters of this book, through a prospective look at the societal changes underway.

Florence Guignard has worked hard for a psychoanalysis which thinks about and ponders on its continuation, its future, constantly seeking to articulate the concepts stemming from the models of drive functioning, internal object relationships and intersubjective relations.

It becomes clear today, on the occasion of the republication of her *very first* book, how much it incorporates within it the foundations of the conceptions and themes developed in her later works. We find in it models and "psychoanalytic concepts in movement" (Guignard, 2015) which are all the more necessary in order to bring the suffering of contemporary man into contact with the *child of yesteryear* who lives in him forever.

Sesto-Marcello Passone

Chapter 1

The Infantile in the analytic relationship*

The analytic relationship

Every psychoanalyst is aware that his professional specificity is woven from his very identity, because his working instrument is his own psychic structure, even though, being unconscious, it remains almost entirely unknown to itself.

Day by day, therefore, in each encounter with each of his patients, he must take account of and utilize this virtually unknown element, which is in a constant state of flux and can therefore never be permanently grasped by his personal analysis or analyses. Dominated, protected and blinded as it is by both primary and secondary repression, the analyst must nevertheless commit his psychic structure without restriction to his daily task; while the processes of this structure are essentially unconscious, bearing witness to and containing the repressed past, they also constitute a reservoir of hitherto merely latent forms and drive energy that can be drawn upon for his cathexes, whether narcissistic or of objects.

When confronted with so much that is inexpressible, the human mind cannot but seek to get its bearings by trying out representations and metaphors, but this carries the risk of freezing a particular configuration like a snapshot. While not wishing to begin by imposing a fixed pattern on my presentation, I should like to compare the analytic encounter to a constantly moving, variable-geometry constellation of impact points that generate tensions between two virtual loci which can be imagined as two psychic spaces, the analyst's and the analysand's, each having its own organization.

As a metaphor of a two-fold fiction, figurative cut-outs of something that remains unknowable in itself, these boundary meeting-places are accessible to the mind only by representation and symbolization. Yet they will be required to assume a functional role: having been explored by the analyst through his personal analysis, they will be cathected by the analysand on the model of his past relationships, i.e. in the *transference.* In the analyst these are the loci where both his *countertransference* and his *valence as an anaclitic object* arise, whereas in the analysand they will be the sites where the cathexis of the neurotic *repetition* is reoriented towards *remembering* and the preconditions for *working-through.*

This working-through will, of course, be based on the specific *logic of the unconscious,* whose characteristics, as described by Freud (1915c) and developed in particular by Bion (1961), Matte Blanco (1975) and Neyraut (1978), are as follows:

1 The logic of the unconscious knows no contradiction, so that there is no negation.
2 It treats asymmetrical relationships as if they were symmetrical, so that seriation in time and space does not exist.
3 It knows nothing of the organizational and hierarchical configurations whereby the part is connected with the whole and the beginning with the end, so that it operates in infinite loops.
4 It works simultaneously with the logic of the system *Cs.*, so that a field of tensions and interactions analogous to the field of activity linking unconscious fantasies with the thought mode of dreams arises between the two logics.

Among the elements of the elaborative work that will continue in analyst and analysand alike as long as the treatment lasts, I wish to lay particular emphasis on the configuration of the process in the here-and-now of the session whereby repression is lifted or certain splits may be modified within the representations of the analytic relationship.

This process will after all facilitate the emergence of derivatives of representations of the current state of the intrapsychic conflict in the system *Pcs.* of one or the other, or preferably both, of the two protagonists of the treatment.

We have been accustomed to think that the asymmetry of the two parties has a dynamizing effect, owing to the high value that we as analysts place on our long personal analysis and the presumed permanent self-analysis that follows it. However, analytic activity inherently sets many traps for the unwary, so that this asymmetry may not infrequently also blind the analyst. The requirement of so-called "evenly suspended" attention admittedly entails a state of mind that encourages the permeability of the repression barrier. Yet we are familiar from our day-to-day practice with the resistances to the establishment and maintenance of this kind of attention. They are due to the coalescence of transference/countertransference factors connected with the limits of the two protagonists' psychic capacities and they ally themselves with each party's unconscious representations, whose preconscious derivatives it is the job of the analyst to observe in himself.

A basic mode and rhythm proper to each analytic relationship arises in the normal course of a treatment, and the analyst learns to observe the particular tone assumed by the process.

This original and specific rhythm may, however, be disrupted. Again, because it is analogous to the rhythms of respiration or circulation, minor disturbances to it may well be denied. More significant disturbances are commonly attributed to the *transference*. But they may also be regarded as *blind spots in the countertransference*, which have caught the analyst unawares.

The point, however, is that in a "well-tempered" conflictual configuration, *any break in communication will be reflected by a representational deficiency*. Both the analyst and the analysand unconsciously experience this deficiency as the *loss of a significant internal object* – no matter whether good or bad – and it will normally set in train an unconscious process of figuration akin to dreaming with the same vicissitudes. Like a dream, this process will in most cases instantly be swallowed up by repression. Sometimes it will take the form of a confused upsurge of images accompanied by loss of the boundaries between self and other, between outside and inside and between perception and hallucination – unless, in the most favourable case, a combined word-and thing-presentation offers itself to the analytic work of association and decondensation.

However partial and ephemeral, the use of representations offered by a third party – whether internal, in the form of the analyst's reverie or even his writing, or external, through a colleague – generally has an illuminating effect, helping to make the analyst once again available to his patient's analytic process. The analyst must also have acquired a certain discipline of thought if he is to have any chance of noticing this deficiency. The bipolar concepts of Bion (1963) and Green's (1993) important contribution on the negative in psychic functioning ought to have penetrated sufficiently deeply into our thinking to allow us to demand more rigorous analytic performance from ourselves as it were by deferred action after the deployment of evenly suspended attention during the session.

By thus reflecting on our day-to-day mode of functioning, I have developed an approach that has for some time now underlain my attempts to grasp the basic elements that seem to me to be concerned in the functioning of the analytic relationship. I believe that a recent contribution of mine (Guignard, 1994a) represents a significant advance in this respect. It discusses the historical reasons why the reference to the child and the Infantile-in-the-adult will in my view always be indispensable in both clinical psychoanalysis and metapsychology; and it contains two metapsychological hypotheses that I used to examine the theoretical and technical aspects of the subject with specific reference to the countertransference.

I should now like to return to the place of the Infantile in the analytic relationship, with a view to making further hypotheses on its role in the psychoanalyst's functioning in the session.

The Infantile in the adult

For all the variation of the concept from author to author and between different contributions by one and the same author, the explicit or implicit reference to "the child" and "the Infantile" permeates the whole of the psychoanalytic literature, starting with Freud. Before putting forward my personal view, I shall give some examples of the omnipresence of the Infantile in Freud's work:

1 The discovery of infantile sexuality, involving polymorphous perversion and the vicissitudes of the establishment of an economy between the pleasure/unpleasure principle and the reality principle, a process initiated by the activation of a field mobilizing both hallucination and perception.
2 The discovery of early unconscious psychic functioning, which gives rise on the one hand to psychic contents and on the other to a repressing agency that will operate throughout life on two simultaneous levels, primary and secondary.
3 The organization of mental life, from the very first sensory relations and the first motor actions on the subject's own body and on objects in external reality, accompanied in the system *Pcs.* by the establishment of the twin spirals of (i) the primary and secondary processes that constitute the matrix of fantasy life, and (ii) the processes of symbolization.
4 The Oedipal organization, which is specific to the human species, with its different levels of complexity, on the one hand relational and objectifying and on the other narcissistic and identificatory.
5 The containing framework of this Oedipal organization, conceptualized as a psychic space, allowing the free exchange of intrapsychic conflicts between the three agencies of the id, the ego and the superego.
6 The infantile neurosis as the basic model both of psychopathology and of the therapeutic situation, in the form of its homologue, the transference neurosis, in which the fixation points and the defence mechanism of regression give rise to constant circulation between past and present, between infantile and adult forms of cathexis and thought.

I therefore wish to shift the emphasis even further from the subjective towards the intersubjective and from metaphor to conceptualization, from the analyst to the analytic relationship and from the child to the Infantile. This will modify the symbolic level of my parameters and call for some new definitions.

Brusset (1994, p. 705) – in particular his conclusion that "the Infantile as a category of psychic causality lies in an intermediate position between the unconscious outside time and the individual childhood history", strikes an immediate chord in me; however, owing to the novelty of my own conceptualization of the Infantile, I feel justified in taking the following step-by-step approach to its definition:

As a strange historical/ahistorical conglomerate, the crucible of primal fantasies and sensorimotor experiences that can be stored as memory traces, the Infantile may be regarded as the psychic locus of the first unrepresentable emergences of the drives. All that we can ever know of this "advanced action" is its representable derivatives, in the form of infantile sexual theories on the one hand and memory traces on the other.

The Infantile is a basic structure on the fringes of our animal nature, the depository and container of our drives, be they libidinal or hateful on the one hand or epistemophilic on the other. It is that combination of drive-related and flexible structural elements that makes a person who he is and not someone else. Irreducible, unique and hence universal, the Infantile is therefore the entity that will usher in our mental life, through all the developments of its psychic bisexuality as organized by the Oedipus complex.

A psychic place of primary and unrepresentable drive emergences on the boundary of the *Ucs.* and *Pcs.*, the Infantile is the culminating point of our affects, the locus of hope and of cruelty, of courage and unconcern; it operates throughout life, in a twin spiral of process and assignment of meaning, and can even be discerned in the most severe pathologies, provided that these are not confused with its normal mode of organization.

And if the Infantile in us continues until our dying day to operate simultaneously at the level of secondary Oedipal processes and of primitive mechanisms, this is because it partakes of the astonishing force of the drives, the fantastic unfolding of which can be observed in the rhythm of psychic development at the very beginning of human life.

However, the drive element is not the only entity involved in this attempt to define the Infantile. In its metaphorical aspect, the concept also applies to its hallucinatory and protosymbolic retinue of preforms that are constantly evolving in all our mental activities. Once the fixation points that freeze our modes of being and of having in sterile repetition are released by analytic treatment, these preforms will restore the vigour and underlying drive energy to more mature organizations, setting the tone for our individual personality in its normal adult functioning.

My theoretical and technical discussion of the Infantile in the analytic relationship will therefore embrace different levels and will be based on two complementary hypotheses.

1 The first concerns the nature, situation and consequences of the points of impact of the Infantile-in-the-analysand on the psychoanalyst's mental functioning.

2 The second has to do with the very particular status of the psychoanalyst in relation to the termination criteria of his own analysis and to the post-analytic modifications of his own repressed infantile elements that allow him to function professionally.

Impact of the Infantile-in-the-analysand on the psychoanalyst

Many aspects of the Infantile-in-the-analysand may impact on the psychoanalyst's mental functioning, but the following are perhaps the most relevant to my first hypothesis:

1 The density of the infantile drive organization and the paradoxical expression of the analysand's cathexes in the transference as reflected in the here-and-now of the session.
2 The pressure of the individual analysand's infantile relational and identificatory history on his mode of cathecting fantasy life and external stimuli and on his capacity to differentiate between the two.
3 His different modes of infantile thought, attached in the transference neurosis to the fixation points of his infantile neurosis, and coupled in most cases with traumatic and transgenerational factors.

I therefore postulate that the effect of the Infantile-in-the-other on any subject, even if he is analysed and a psychoanalyst to boot, gives rise to unbound excitation owing to the drive force thereby released. The excitation aroused by the Infantile-in-the-other in my view impinges on the system *Pcs.*; it generates blind spots when it encounters either unanalysed infantile aspects of the recipient or current drive-related derivatives of his unconscious, which by definition arise spontaneously in infantile form.

The normal fate of the excitation aroused in any subject by the Infantile-in-the-other is diversification: on the one hand it is bound by sublimation while on the other it undergoes a fresh repression as a protective shield against stimuli in interpersonal relations. Furthermore, although a linear psychogenetic view might suggest otherwise, I consider that the problem will not be tackled by secondary repression alone. The drive excitation will also trigger a response from the first defensive system, organized around primary repression, while the task of secondary repression will be to back up this first level of defences by the intervention of a post-Oedipal superego.

The same should apply to the psychoanalyst at work. However, his intrapsychic countertransference conflict situation is more complex, because he is in the paradoxical situation of having to direct his attention precisely towards what presents itself to him as a blind spot, generated by the encounter within him between two heterogeneous manifestations of the Infantile: the analysand's transference projection and his own countertransference.

The qualities and characteristics of the Infantile-in-the-psychoanalyst are bound to play a vital part in the relational and identificatory process that stems from the regularity and duration of the several-times-a-week analytic encounters with the qualities and characteristics of the specific-infantile-of-a-specific-analysand. The importance of these qualities will emerge in the use or otherwise made by the analyst of the excitation blind spot due to the Infantile-in-the-analysand for his personal narcissistic and drive-related purposes.

I contend that this blind spot denotes the field of tension generated in the analyst's system *Pcs.* by the excitation; starting from an impulse to fulfil the wish, this field may have one component whereby the wish is repressed and another that becomes a framing and containing preform for the treatment of the relevant analysand. The psychoanalyst's preconscious functioning will therefore determine whether the outcome is acting out, resulting in destruction of the analytic situation, or repression so that the work of analysis is wasted and fails to evolve as it might otherwise have done or, finally, the turning to account of this renewed acquaintance with the Infantile in self and other for framing and containing purposes in aid of what Green (1983) would call life narcissism.

Termination criteria of the psychoanalyst's analysis and the particular status of his repression

This sketch of the situation of the Infantile in the psychoanalyst at work leads on quite naturally to my second hypothesis, which is that the psychoanalyst is in a very particular position with regard to the termination criteria of his own analysis and to post-analytic adaptations of the repression of the Infantile in him as required by the demands of his professional work.

All analysts would no doubt agree that a psychoanalyst-to-be must have undergone a sufficiently deep and detailed personal analysis to enable him to listen without the need to mobilize defences that might obstruct the ongoing process in his analysands; in particular, he should be able to dispense with projective defences and the course of his own associations should not be disrupted by inhibitions.

I would, however, argue that these considerations do not yet tell us anything about the status of the Infantile in the day-to-day functioning of the psychoanalyst. I am not thinking only of the factors which had previously caused his own infantile neurosis, defined as the prevalence of an Oedipal organization, whether or not pathological, in an individual's psychic functioning. On that level, even if we have ultimately had to acknowledge that the infantile neurosis can never be totally "dissolved" as Freud had hoped, we are nevertheless entitled to expect the analytic process to induce a genuine economic or even structural modification, so that the phrase "resolution of the transference neurosis" remains meaningful, if only relatively, when applied to non-psychotic patients.

I see the Infantile here more as the lifelong matrix for the entry of the drives into psychic life, conferring density and complexity on the object relations of every human being whether analysed or not, and at the same time colouring conceptual thought with primary fantasies through the intermediary of unconscious infantile sexual theories.

Five points may be made concerning this problem:

1 When a neurotic formation is resolved through analytic work, this does not necessarily mean that the drive-based, relational and identificatory elements caught up in it have also been disposed of. On the contrary, they are likely to be liberated; some will be adapted and recathected in modified narcissistic and object configurations, while others will undergo a fresh repression, albeit less disabling because more appropriate than its predecessor.
2 For the psychoanalyst at work, one of the essential new cathexes accruing from his personal analysis is his ability to make more appropriate use of the boundaries of his ego as a container for the Infantile in himself. As an antidote to the pathological overflowing of narcissism, this capacity reduces the risk of the psychoanalyst's being seduced and led by this child-in-himself. The characteristics of the Infantile, which seeks to impose the omniscience and omnipotence of "His Majesty the baby", must after all be taken into account. If this omniscience is allowed to hold sway, the psychoanalyst might end up including his analysand in a narcissistic reflection, to which he might then apply projective interpretations; in this case, his omnipotence might cause him to act out in the countertransference.
3 By definition, repression takes control of anything connected with the drives, the Infantile, the traumatic and the pathology of internal objects (objects-of-internal-objects and transgenerational problems). For this reason, the new post-analytic repression in the psychoanalyst will draw into its wake not only the aspects of the Infantile in himself that did not find expression or remained unanalysed in his own analysis, but also what I shall call the basic components of his *Weltanschauung*. These comprise in particular his infantile sexual theories, as defensive manifestations of his primal fantasies, and his screen memories. Freud even contended that the familiar childhood amnesia, which is theoretically so important to us, is completely counterbalanced by screen memories: "They represent the forgotten years of childhood as adequately as the manifest content of a dream represents the dream-thoughts" (Freud, 1914, p. 148).

4 The importance of the Infantile in the psychoanalyst's mental functioning may appear self-evident, but the psychic economy of the situation is actually far from simple. This is because it presupposes that the analyst at work is constantly combating his normal post-analytic repression, that is, what could be called the "tertiary" repression of much of the infantile in himself that have been liberated from their neurotic organization.

The excitation bound up with the drive force of the Infantile-in-the-analyst will therefore be artificially diverted from a part of its fate – i.e. repression – so that the analyst can use it in his work. There may thus be a contradiction in our criteria for the termination or continuation of candidates' analyses.

5 This brings us back to the issue of analysis terminable or interminable raised by Freud:

> It seems that a number of analysts learn to make use of defensive mechanisms which allow them to divert the implications and demands of analysis from themselves (probably by directing them on to other people), so that they themselves remain as they are and are able to withdraw from the critical and corrective influence of analysis. . . . It would not be surprising if the effect of a constant preoccupation with all the repressed material which struggles for freedom in the human mind were to stir up in the analyst as well all the instinctual demands which he is otherwise unable to keep under suppression.
>
> (Freud, 1937, p. 249)

Freud, it will be recalled, goes on to advise the analyst to resubmit himself to analysis every five years – a periodicity which cannot but put us in mind of the age of the Oedipus complex. He concludes: "This would mean, then, that not only the therapeutic analysis of patients but his own analysis would change from a terminable into an interminable task" (ibid.).

Infantile illnesses in the counter transference

It will be noted that, in considering the analytic relationship from the point of view of the Infantile, I am taking care not to present yet another aetiological hypothesis on the wide-ranging question about "becoming a psychoanalyst". I am confining myself to a reflexive observation on the functioning of an "infantile" that must be cathected particularly strongly and permanently by a psychoanalyst if he is to be able to listen adequately to his analysand's infantile neurosis.

I am therefore asking "how" rather than "why" and would argue as follows:

1 As we have seen, in impacting on the system *Pcs.* of the other, the Infantile-in-the-adult gives rise to an excitation that both carries within itself and generates Oedipal movements and primal fantasies. For this reason, at least in neurotic-normal functioning, this excitation and its twin retinue usually undergo a repression whose nature and quality will determine the forms of the return of the repressed, which may range from acts to thought.
2 We are familiar with the classical normal exceptions to this rule, namely, the state of being in love, the normal illness of the mother with her capacity for reverie, and the transference relationship.
3 It seems to me to follow from my remarks on the Infantile-in-the-psychoanalyst that because of the countertransference work the analyst must, in his analytic listening, *artificially stop the normal process of repression from affecting the impact of the excitation on his system Pcs. by the Infantile-in-the-analysand.* The countertransference relationship would then be another normal exception. Apart from any infantile conflicts that may have escaped the analyst's personal analysis, we may think of this professional requirement of constantly listening out for the point where drive elements enter the psychic field as a particular modality of the termination criteria of the psychoanalyst's analysis, connected with the status of the Infantile-in-the-analyst, which is thus experimentally kept as close as possible to consciousness.
4 We examine our analysands' words for indications of our parental role in the transference, and may take it for granted that we experience that role identically in the countertransference. However, we may perfectly well be wrong in this assumption, as I shall illustrate by the following virtually classical paradigm.

A severe and rigid post-Oedipal parental superego often constitutes the manifest aspect of the imagos projected by the analysand on to the analyst, but in our interpretive choices we must also take account of the simultaneous projection on to us of the complementary latent imago, that of a weak ego, whose infantile impotence is denied by its opposite, infantile omnipotence. The latter will make a seductive narcissistic appeal to its homologue, the infantile omnipotence of the analyst, whose countertransference position in terms of his management of his analysand's superego projection may in turn be influenced by it.

In other words, the conflictual projection of analysands' infantile neurosis on to the adult structures of the analyst entails a constant risk of collusion of the Infantile-in-the-patient with the Infantile-in-the-analyst, at the point of impact of the former on the analyst's system *Pcs.*

If it goes unnoticed, this excitatory point of impact forms a blind spot and tends to be repressed before the analyst has subjected it to self-analysis. It is then liable to resurface in acting out in the countertransference; alternatively, if it is displaced outside the analytic relationship, the analyst may act out in his personal life or suffer somatic effects.

But if the analyst is sufficiently interested in, and attentive to, the Infantile activated in him by the analysand, the same excitation may allow him to generate the preform mentioned earlier, which acts specifically as a protective shield against stimuli and container for the infantile elements in the transference/countertransference relationship.

The difference between the sexes and the generations in the working through of the Oedipus complex is of course constantly and repeatedly called into question at every instant of our working day as psychoanalysts. Our attention to this model, which I see as a dynamizing element of the intrapsychic conflict in the transference-countertransference relationship, may therefore enable us to discover and analyse a whole set of interactions, which are active although latent, between the Infantile-in-the-analysand and the Infantile-in-the-psychoanalyst.

These essentially narcissistic phenomena underlying the manifest parental transferences that we are more accustomed to look for play their silent parts in the respective primal scenes of the analysand and the analyst in the succession of transference and countertransference identifications. In the guise of the mirror relationship, of the situation of the double, and of mimetic identification, the economy and dynamics of the exchanges between the Infantile in the two protagonists may also extend to bisexual complementarity or to the child's parental or therapeutic function, as well as to jealousy, rivalry, incest and murder in the transference and countertransference alike.

These subtle and complex unconscious exchanges occur in the space which Freud (1905) had already characterized in the *Three Essays on the Theory of Sexuality* , that is to say, on the boundaries of polymorphism and of perversion. They therefore inevitably affect the development and equilibrium of the psychic lives of both partners in the analytic treatment.

Traps set by the Infantile for the psychoanalyst's functioning in the session

What effects do these matters have on the functioning of the psychoanalyst in the session and in particular on his interpretive activity?

I shall approach this question from the point of view of the *negative,* which is for me the *category to which the blind spots arising from the impact of the Infantile-in-the-analysand on the analyst's preconscious system belong*. I postulated earlier that every blind spot is reflected in a representational deficiency in the transference-countertransference communication, and that this deficiency is experienced as the loss of a significant object. I noted that this loss sets in train a process of figuration at unconscious level that is akin to dreaming and suffers the same fate: repression, blurring of the boundaries between perception and hallucination, or emergence of a representation.

However, the unconscious malaise arising from this deficiency induces not only the analysand but also the analyst to deny it as far as possible. There then arise the kind of pseudo-associations that I have called *stopper-representations,* intended to camouflage the silent haemorrhage of libido and objects in the relational field between the analyst and the analysand.

As long as they occur in the analysand, these unmeaningful representations are relatively easy for an experienced analyst to detect. They are much more insidious and difficult to get rid of when they arise in the analyst, because his basic cultural object – that is to say, his corpus of theory – is then shamelessly swallowed up in this unexpected chasm, with all the ensuing advantages and disadvantages characteristic of "group mentality" (Bion, 1961).

In my opinion, the impact of the Infantile-in-the-analysand on the system *Pcs.* of the psychoanalyst is an occasion *par excellence* for such a situation. The analyst's functioning will then "go down a notch", as he abandons the anguish of uncertainty and of the position "without memory or desire" (Bion, 1970) and falls back on the allegedly obvious. We will now observe the stock reflex actions of our trade, the most common of which are:

1 References to the analysand's personal history.
2 Psychoanalytic theory.
3 Blaming the analysand.

1 *The analysand's personal history* is widely resorted to, especially if it includes one or more apparently severe traumas. Repeated references to an event in the analysand's history deemed significant by the analyst will act as a *stopper-representation* in the precise position of *the blind spot denoting the meeting place of the Infantiles of the analysand and of the analyst;* this repetition will thus prevent full – i.e. transferential – analysis of the psychic trauma. This use of event-related material is to my mind hysterical in nature and has the effect, if not the unconscious aim, in the analyst of maintaining a degree of unbound drive excitation in the transference – countertransference field, thereby repetitively eroticizing this field on an infantile level – specifically, a sadomasochistic one – to the detriment of any thought activity.

Now an analysand who regularly hears most of the elements of his dreams and associations referred to the account he has tried to give of his past will eventually discover that this is how his analyst defends himself. However much the latter brings him back to instances of abandonment by important figures in his childhood, the analysand will not be fooled forever by the analyst's phobia about the Infantile in himself. So, the insidious attacks on the analytic process will persist.

2 As everyone knows, *recourse to psychoanalytic theory* was one of the foibles of the inventor of psychoanalysis. We are all familiar with the temptation to do likewise, with the obvious aim of avoiding something painful in the emotional field of the analytic relationship. In my opinion, the blind spot caused by the impact on the analyst of the Infantile-in-the-analysand is particularly likely to result in the use of *psychoanalytic theory as a stopper-representation.*

This was the case, for example, with *infantile sexual theories*, a catch-all concept embracing both drive and defence. Freud's (1909) *discovery of infantile sexuality* was both a breakthrough and a *defence*, protecting him from the outrageousness of his own discovery. By remaining at the manifest pregenital level of his theories, he minimized the scandal of infantile sexuality, which, of course, lies in the earliness of its genital component. At the same time he camouflaged the perspicacity demonstrated by Little Hans' raptures over the beauty of his newborn sister's widdler. It is this element of infantile genitality that the Professor was unable to integrate into his theories, instead seizing without hesitation on all the defensive "unisex" comments made by the "little investigator".

It is hardly necessary to add that, even without his genius, we are no less defensive today than Freud was in the past and that, more often than we ought, we confuse the stopper-representations that infantile sexual theories by definition are with the living psychic reality of the child or adult. Thierry Bokanowski (1996) tackles the problem with particular reference to the conflicts – which may be either fruitful or destructive according to the circumstances – between "*the child theorist* within [the analyst] and certain unconscious derivatives of the *infantile sexual theories* put to him by his patient" (p. 161). He describes the psychoanalyst's experience as falling within the category of the uncanny and even postulates a "bedrock of denial of the Infantile".

3 *Blaming the analysand* as if he were a dunce for refusing to understand an interpretation that was perfectly clear and repeated unsuccessfully several times ought to represent the ultimate alarm system for any psychoanalyst on the lookout for his blind spots.

This expedient unfortunately plays no small part in the delicate psychic economy of such a practitioner, who must all day receive and accept projections, most of which are to say the least unpleasant. He will therefore be subject to a powerful unconscious temptation either artificially to give a "stopper-interpretation" or to arouse in the analysand a "stopper representation", in the deceptive guise of an all-purpose, "What do you think of it?"

Sometimes it is the analysand who expresses the situation best, when he complains at this precise time that he no longer feels held and contained by the analytic situation. Because the analyst was unaware of his own blind spot, it has not been possible for the underlying drive excitation generated by the encounter between the two "Infantiles" to be transformed into a psychically representable conflict. The analytic material thus remains in a fuzzy, ill-defined state in which it cannot be represented, and hence repressed, although it exists in the form of drive pressure on the analyst's system *Pcs.*

This situation would merely constitute a waste of the analysand's money and of both protagonists' time – although that too is by no means negligible – were it not for the fact that it severely burdens the analysand with the analyst's unconscious guilt about his own blind spot. From then on repetition of the past, with its retinue of both primary and secondary defences, will be uppermost in the analytic relationship.

In order to define the Infantile and examine its role in the analytic relationship, I have considered its developmental as well as its structural aspects. My position is supported both by Freud's dual conception of the unconscious as constituting not only a container for the repressed but also a reservoir of drives, and by the spontaneous combination of the two Freudian models of the psychic apparatus, which are neither mutually exclusive nor always easy to use together.

This led me to consider the specific criteria for termination of the analyst's analysis and the economic situation of repression in the psychoanalyst at work.

In characterizing the impact of the Infantile-in-the-analysand on the psychoanalyst's system *Pcs.* from both the narcissistic and the relational viewpoint, I discussed the vicissitudes of the representational deficiency and attempted to examine the status and fate of the blind spots aroused by that impact. Involving as it does the negative, work on such blind spots seems to bear some relation to post-traumatic or indeed post-hypnotic situations, as Green (1993) remarks about a hypnotic subject's putting up his umbrella for no reason long after emerging from hypnosis. He notes that the performance in fact demonstrated not so much the unconscious of the impressionable and suggestible subject as the suggestive force of the hypnotist. The author points out that the work of the negative could be *inferred* from the second phase of the operation, the hypnotized subject's rationalization when answering the question, "Why did you put up your umbrella?": The object of the answer "To see if it works" is surely intended to obliterate the hypnotist's subjectivity by the assertion of the subject's own subjectivity, thus breaking the link joining the couple involved in the experience and leaving room only for the will of the subject.

The blind spot is an expression of the analyst's denial of the fantasy of seduction by the analysand's infantile omnipotence, and as such is a narcissistic defence whose unconscious aim is to break the link joining the couple involved in the experience by a kind of phallic outbidding along the lines of: "I respond to your omnipotence with omnipotence and a half!"

At this point the fate of the analyst condemned to fight against his normal repression may prove advantageous: the more he is compelled to remember the penury of identity camouflaged by omnipotence, the easier it will be for him to discover the primal fantasies that lie behind his defensive phallic infantile sexual theory and to use his psychic bisexuality in his communication with the analysand, on the founding level of the Oedipus complex and of the primal scene.

Note

* This chapter was first published in *International Journal of Psycho-Analysis*, 1995, 76, pp. 1083–1093 (Guignard, 1995a). It was translated by Philip Slotkin and has been very slightly modified for this edition.

Chapter 2

Hans and Sigi

Sexual theories as defences against the discovery of infantile sexuality

The thirst for knowledge and its entropy

I want to offer here some reflections concerning the relationships between the organization of thought and its drive-related and identificatory foundations. The thirst for knowledge, the avowed profession of faith of any researcher, cannot be conceived without its complement, which I would call entropic: the *danger of knowing*. The conflict between these two tendencies manifests itself in various ways, in particular by the tendency on the one hand to fall into a Manichean dichotomy and, on the other, to operate trivial repressions. So we separate the body from the mind, the visible from the invisible, the expressible from the inexpressible, and the measurable from the immeasurable.

Thus, when Freud revealed the scandal of infantile sexuality to the world, he could not avoid unconsciously repeating part of his own repression of this scandalous sexuality, making sublimation the heir of pregenital impulses alone. It was as if he had shrunk from the most incredible implications of the consequences of his discovery: the affirmation of the existence of genital impulses in children, at an age when they are far from being able to fulfil their biological procreative destiny, and the part played by this genitality in all truly creative work.

From the multidisciplinary research that I directed and carried out (Guignard, 1972) many years ago on the subject of children suffering from a mild intellectual impairment, I have drawn two lines of reflection:

1 Such an impairment can serve as a bulwark, albeit sometimes fragile, against a delusional schizophrenic psychopathology, as was developed later in one of our subjects. In other words, some of these children are dumb to avoid being crazy. The crumbling of the ego seems to act as an interface between the schizophrenia of the young adult and a state of health precariously maintained by stupidity so as not to fall into madness.

2 The poverty of fantasy activity during the latency period in children with an otherwise normal IQ is undoubtedly a serious pathological indicator, contrary to what we can read in the classic literature. Indeed, this deficiency in fantasy activity during the period of latency is the expression of the defensive foundations of severe infantile neuroses that can be observed later in adults. Something has "castrated" the thirst for knowledge in these children.

The "foolishness" of Little Hans and the guilt of Little Sigi

I propose to study some of these processes with regard to Little Hans. Indeed, contrary to Freud (1909, p. 27) who, in the study of this case, affirms that "a neurosis never says foolish things", I think that it is in the very logic of Freudian discoveries on the conflictual dynamics of the drives with their vicissitudes to consider the neurosis as a "corner of foolishness" in the organization of the subject.

As we will see with Leonardo da Vinci, and although Freud very clearly linked Little Hans' inquisitiveness – "this little investigator" as he calls him – to the development of his Oedipus complex, he did not give the thirst for knowledge the status of a metapsychological concept. By repeating it repeatedly within the framework of curiosity about the origins and in connection with the birth, feared or proven, of another child, Freud seems to me to invoke the coherence of his theoretical system to hide the personal trauma that the brief existence of his brother Julius represented for him. Ernest Jones (1953–1957, my emphasis) writes on this subject:

> he had to learn from experience how strong the jealousy of a young a child can be. In a letter to Fliess, in 1897, he admits the evil wishes he had against his rival and adds that their fulfillment in his death had aroused self-reproaches, *a tendency that had remained ever since.*
>
> (in Masson, 1985, p. 8, my emphasis)

It is commonplace to note that the story of Freud's countertransference towards Hans is complex:

1 The story was told to him by the father of the child, who was one of his pupils.
2 Freud had had Hans' mother in analysis some time before.
3 The personal equation of his relationship with his own mother seems to have played an important role in his way of listening to what was said to him about Little Hans' sexual curiosity and fantasies about the difference between the sexes.

It was in this very particular context of repeating his own Oedipal situation that Freud chose to retain as the so-called universal sexual theory only the ultimate and very well-known unisex version that Hans – in desperation, I might say – gave his mother: "I thought that you were so tall that you'd have a widdler like a horse" (Freud, 1909, p. 10).

Yet several months earlier, even though Hans' mother had recently been pregnant with Hanna, the father had reported to Freud the following dialogue: "Mummy, have you got a widdler too?" To which his mother replied: "Of course.[1] Why?" And Hans said, thoughtfully: "I was only just thinking" (ibid., p. 7).

If we recall that Hans was exposed to a great deal of bodily intimacy with his mother who got dressed in front of him and let him enter the bathroom with her, the three accounts of this story – from mother to father, then from father to Freud and finally from Freud to his readers – makes all the protagonists of the scene lose much of their innocence:

1 Did not Hans, as all children do, spread the lie in order to know if he was allowed to speak the truth about the difference of the sexes – rather than about the absence of his mother's widdler?
2 Did not the mother, enjoying being flirtatious, eroticize the situation, both with her little boy and with her husband and, above all, with her ex-analyst, to whom she knew the story would be faithfully transmitted?
3 Did not the father, through an impulse of infantile transference rivalry with his wife and son with regard to Freud, unconsciously seek to assert himself homosexually in the eyes of the master by means of his virile adult attributes?
4 As for Freud, did he not have some Oedipal and countertransference reasons for denying, through the interpretation he gave of Hans' remarks, his own desire for his mother's genitals as well as those of this woman who had been his patient?

Zonal confusion and entropy of intuitive knowledge

Sexual theories admittedly proceed from a certain degree of zonal confusion, as evidenced by the cloacal hypothesis. Now I would like to put forward the idea that these confusions constitute a defensive formation, which coexists with a certain degree of unconscious knowledge of sexual differences, knowledge stemming from the perceptual visual and proprioceptive activity of the child. These confusions are used by the child defensively whenever his desire comes into conflict with external reality and with the requirements of his internal objects, of which the very first is the superego. However, the age at which Hans allegedly had this conversation with his pregnant mother is precisely the age when "genital impulses" – Freud also tells us – are at their peak. Is it any wonder, then, that the child was particularly sensitive to the atmosphere of sexual excitation which surrounded him and for which he was not solely responsible?

Unfortunately, he seems to have paid the price and, without going so far as to attribute the development of his phobia to these factors alone, I would like to highlight what, in the sexual excitation of the adults around him, certainly must have represented a considerable danger to him in the pursuit of his epistemophilic investigations.

First of all, by avoiding communicating verbally with her son about a reality – her female genitals – the entry of which she had given him many opportunities of perceiving, Hans' mother exhibited magical genitals, whose obviousness – *selbstverständlich* – was only matched by their ambiguity, as evidenced by Hans' suspended response: "I was only just thinking". The little boy felt both castrated by his thirst for knowledge, which had suddenly been forbidden, and cheated in the confidence he had in his mother by the equivocal answer which substituted for the genital difference of the sexes the pregenital aspect of the question – every human being has a urinary tract, therefore a "widdler" (*Wiwi-macher*). From then on, Hans' love for his mother came into conflict with his thirst for knowledge, which she treated in the mode of a symbolic equation as an incestuous desire.

The pseudo-silly remark that he made some time later about a cow that was being milked – "Oh, look! There's milk coming out of its widdler" (p. 7) – painfully evokes, in this little boy who was otherwise so bright, the existence of a need for conformity that exists in an endemic state in cases of endogenous intellectual impairment. Indeed, clinical experience shows us that the need for love prevails over any developmental impulse from the moment a young child feels that he has lost communication with his primordial objects. He is then able to utter the worst kinds of nonsense, like Hans who, in this example, sacrifices his acute spirit of observation to the mimetic imitation of his mother's *selbstverständlich*: if everyone has a "widdler", the "widdler" can be used for anything and everything, and the symbolic equation can serve as a symbol.

Sadistic conformism in adults as a defence against the perception of the Infantile

But the worst is yet to come in the realm of unconscious sadism. Contrary to what we are told in the manifest discourse of the text, his entourage actually responded to the questions of Little Hans – who, however, carefully disguises them – with silence and avoidance. I'm talking about the story of his mother giving birth. We are told simultaneously that Hans submitted in a completely conformist way – conformism which I see as a defence – to the ambient double discourse to the effect that, first, it was the stork-doctor who brought the baby, and second, that Hans was not spared any of his mother's screams during childbirth. Nobody seemed to understand Hans' pathetic efforts to contain and reassure himself by using, for lack of anything better, the family system of lies to speak about, while at the same time denying it, the frightening perception of his mother's screams: "Mummy's coughing" he said, rather than having an outburst of anxiety. This is a remarkable example of the occasional distortion of perceptual activity, which, in children with intellectual impairments, has become the rule. It was in this connection that more acute attention from the analyst would have been welcome, and one cannot help wondering if Julius had not obliterated Freud's attention, which was so subtle in other circumstances.

Then Hans was brought into the room after the delivery even though there were still basins full of blood and water. It does not seem very surprising to me that, in these distressing conditions, Hans chose the lesser of two evils and that, after apparently ignoring his mother and the new baby – this is not explained to us, although it is the crux of the problem – he exclaimed on seeing the basins: "But blood doesn't come out of *my* widdler!" (p. 10).

We are in a situation of extreme complexity here. Whilst it is common observation that little boys cling to their penis – a representative of their ego – in situations of insecurity, it should be recalled that Hans had been directly threatened with castration if he engaged in any such activity. He appeared to have obeyed this ban by showing himself capable of turning action into words, which led him to talk a lot about his "widdler". However, at this stage in his history, his verbalization resulted all those around him – Freud included – showing increased erotic interest in the remarks he made about this famous "widdler". A hyper-cathexis of this "widdler-talk", caused by impulses that were not his own, led Hans to turn it into a fetish object serving both as a means of expressing conflicts that caused him too much anxiety and as a defence against them. When he entered the bedroom where his mother and the new baby were, Hans knew he had lost everything, and most of all, the love of his mother of early childhood. His remark was certainly a denial of his castration-anxiety, but much more a desperate and derisory attempt to avoid, for a little while, the recognition of the irreparable nature of his loss of love.

It was at this crucial point in his life that Hans lacked the support of those around him to help him use his instinctual drive resources to understand what he no longer possessed. In other words, the wish to think took over from the wish to possess his mother and supported the beginnings of a renunciation of his Oedipal object. But it was also at this crucial point that his parents showed maximum blindness, making repeated sadistic errors and projecting their own denial on to the child. This considerably increased Hans' guilt for thinking, and this was when a somatic symptom occurred (sore throat) to which Freud did not give any meaning, any more than he did to the radical castration that resulted from it (tonsillectomy) Now we can suppose that this was his way of experiencing his projective identification with "Mummy's coughing", that is to say, with his mother giving birth, in pain and blood. One may also wonder to what extent all or part of this somatization could have been avoided if some sort of dialogue had been established with Hans. Still, for this to have been effective, it would have been necessary to *sense his wish to understand*, through "Mummy's coughing" rather than taking it as an object of scientific observation or a funny remark.

But childhood amnesia makes the adult a stranger to the child he was. And when, later in life, other children – his own, for example – come to make demands on the repressed in the adult, the latter will defend himself by reprojecting on to the child his own split-off and denied parts, often pervaded by sadism which returns without being either recognized or elaborated. If he is not careful, the adult will tend with any child in possession of language to use a projective mode of communication that is characteristic of a child in the latency period: repression of sexuality, body-psyche split, conformism matched by ostracism, clan spirit based on phallic competition used as denial of the difference of the sexes, primacy of appearances and a concern for "what people will say" over psychic reality, and denigration of expressions of love and affective dependence. One cannot help but think here of the tireless analytical demand that Ferenczi was to address in vain to Freud a few years later. Ferenczi succeeded in using his traumatic experiences to discover several parameters that are essential for theoretical and clinical analysis, such as the trauma/splitting pair on which Bokanowski (1995) has commented so remarkably; but, as we know, somatizations would in the end prematurely take hold of this "wise baby" according to the very law of splitting he had described.

Language of the Infantile

In my assisted listening to the analytic treatments of children, I have many opportunities to reflect on the difficulty adults have in finding authentic contact with the language of the child, and being guided by it in the work of communication in analysis. The child's spontaneous language is more infiltrated by primary processes than is the typical language of the adult; it is woven more with play and action in everyday life and, even more so, in analysis, which helps keep it in close contact with the fantasy-related and representative components of thought processes. As I argued in the first chapter of this book, the *value of sexual excitation* that childish language constitutes for adults is not to be underestimated.

Faced with such seduction, adults will not always have a choice of means to defend themselves: their neurosis will guide their countertransference reactions, which it will be even easier for them to rationalize than in adult treatments, projecting on to the child their own awkward ignorance.

For example, Freud took the trouble to integrate into his account of the treatment the account given by Hans' father of the admiration expressed by the little boy when faced with the whiteness of his father's chest. However, no one seemed to spot, behind this narcissistic admiration for the father, the distress experienced by the child over the loss of his mother's breast – his mother was henceforth devoted to his little sister – and the obvious attempt to displace on to the father a cathexis of the primary maternal object. Here we see the effect of repression at work in the countertransference: *the analyst is unaware that he is reporting material whose meaning he does not understand* – in this case, the homosexual maternal pole of the transference.

If we follow the story of the observation of Little Hans until the outbreak of phobia, we realize that the child had to discover the difference between the sexes in a context of phallocentric fantasy projected on to him, all the feminine attributes being passed over in silence, even in response to his questions. It would take Freud's intervention to restore the situation somewhat, to an extent that he himself considered insufficient. Freud's eroticized countertransference towards Hans' mother and the status of Oedipal rival that Hans' father unconsciously took for him could not be better expressed than in the following passage from the text.

Let's go back to Hans, who we are told "meets everything he sees with a very suspicious and intent look . . . and is very jealous of the new arrival" (Freud, 1909, pp. 10–11). He tries to use his thirst for knowledge to defend himself against the loss of the maternal breast given to the new baby, while expressing his desire to bite both of them:

> [Whenever] anyone praises her, says she is a lovely baby, and so on, etc., he at once declares scornfully: 'But she's not got any teeth yet.' And, in fact, *when he saw her for first time,*[2] he was very much surprised that she was unable to speak, and decided that this was because she had no teeth.
>
> (ibid, p. 11)

We can understand this as a denial: no, it is not this toothless baby who made his mother suffer and scream so much. . .

In the three months following Hanna's birth – Freud's choice of the first name/pseudonym will be appreciated – we can see Hans grappling with the conflict between his thirst for knowledge, whose development, he sensed unconsciously, had been cruelly prohibited by those around him, and anxiety linked to losing his objects of primary love. It may well be, moreover, that most of his parents' Oedipal rivalry with their children, as well as the resulting, more or less explicit, threat of castration, manifested itself essentially in the form of attacks against their child's desire to think, desire that was unconsciously and symbolically equated with the child's sexual desire.

The fact remains that Hans found a *temporary compromise* between his perceptions and the prohibition against naming and recognizing the female genitals: *he thinks the "widdler" is the criterion that distinguishes the animate from the inanimate*. But, contrary to what happens in mentally impaired children, this was not enough to settle the conflict, which reappeared in the form of repeating the same question, this time put to his father: "Daddy, have you got a widdler too?" Here we can see at work the constitutive mechanisms of neurosis, in particular the *progressive condensation* of the conflict in a single element, verbal and/or pictorial, whose ambiguous status Freud later recognized. However, Hans' father gave an identical answer, even in it form, to the one the mother had given to Hans' question: *Selbstverständlich*. Hans pointed out to his father that he had never seen this famous "widdler" when his father was undressing. He then began to doubt his previous perception of his mother who did not hesitate to show him her still unnamed "widdler", whenever she was undressing. Hans' mind was becoming increasingly confused between a paternal "widdler" he was forbidden to see, a maternal "widdler" that was not identified as different from the father's and the son's, and the silence maintained concerning the reasons for the bodily changes in the mother before, during and after her pregnancy – since it was said that it was the stork-doctor (there is more than one paradoxical condensation here) who had brought – or made? – the baby to the mother, who had made her cough and bleed so much.

Identification of the child with the adult mode of defence against infantile sexuality

Hans then tried to find a new solution to the painful conflict situation in which his parents kept him, toying over his questions with their unconscious sadism – stimulated by the situation of the transference on to Freud. He tried to free himself by projecting outside this "widdler" that was clearly too dangerous, the one that had made Mummy cough and bleed and that the tonsillectomy had not permanently remove from inside that part of him traumatically attached to his identification with his mother giving birth. He endowed his mother with an external penis, as big as that of a horse: "I thought you were so big[3] you'd have a widdler like a horse" (Freud, 1909, p. 10). So he could now at least monitor this big *Wiwi-macher* and try to prevent it from bleeding again inside the mother's body and/or his own. This movement of anxiety management was accompanied, as might be expected, by an upsurge in masturbation, an attempt to control both his own desires to penetrate the mother and his terror of the bloody destruction apparently carried out by a penis entering another person's body.

However, this action was not enough to prevent the onset of phobia, the primary form of which was the fear of being bitten by a horse in the street. Hans constructed a "bizarre horse-object" in the sense that (Bion, 1965) gives to "bizarre objects", which I shall describe as a *conglomeration of partial objects and parts of the self, broken up into small parts under the effect of repeated and pathological splitting*. The following forms taken by the phobogenic object are evidence of the same tendencies to form conglomerates: blinkers and black around the mouth of horses, Lizzi's white horse in Gmunden which bites fingers when they are held out to it, etc. It seems important to me to understand that, in this kind of configuration, as in that of delusion, we are no longer dealing with a hidden meaning that needs to be deciphered, but with nonsense, with an *entropy of meaning*.

When Freud (1909, p. 27) declares quite simply that, on the one hand, this cursed phobia, which was resistant to his therapeutic genius, *is not a foolish thing* because "a neurosis never says foolish things, any more than a dream" and, on the other, that Hans' father must tell his son "that this whole story of horses *was a foolish thing* and nothing more", he locks himself into the paradoxical system of nonsense, which serves to prevent real thought from emerging, in the name, I might say, of a mass conformist mentality, that is to say, of Freud's own submission to the basic presuppositions of the socio-cultural group to which he belongs. The consequences of what I think I have identified as an internal conflict in Freud, between the brilliant freedom of thought which was his and this timorous conformism – underpinned, it is true, by the reactivation of his own Oedipal conflict – considerably aggravated Hans' phobia. In fact, Freud was only able to extricate himself from this personal conflict at the cost of acting out that was fraught with consequences: after trying, with the help of Hans' father, to minimize the child's reasons for anxiety, he found nothing better to do than to urge this father to give his son a wild interpretation concerning his sexual desires for his mother and, for good measure, to reaffirm to him that *women and little girls do not have a "widdler", and therefore no genitals*, that reality is unisex and that they are therefore inanimate objects, in keeping with the dichotomy previously established by the child.

In the course of the following months, all sorts of splits can be observed in Hans' mental functioning as well as that of his parents, and it is very fortunate that they – and Freud – really loved this intelligent and endearing little boy. One can scarcely imagine what would have happened to him if this had not been the case, because he would have had to bear the neurosis of his environment as well as his own.

The ignorance of the economic and communication value of Hans' questions in the pre-phobic period may seem astonishing today, especially coming from Freud. It would be comforting to think that advances in analytical technique today protect us from such acting out. I think, alas, that that is not so, having in mind too many current examples of this way of brutally interpreting to patients, both children and adults, their sexual excitation – unless it is perhaps our own? – rather than helping them contain and secondarize it. It is in this precise situation that the analyst's conscious theoretical and technical parameters – and, in particular, the status he grants to the thirst for knowledge – *as well as his split-off and denied infantile sexual theories*, will have an impact on the way he functions. Indeed, these theories guide us at all times, as they guided Freud in his unilateral listening to Little Hans. He wanted to prove that the child spontaneously classifies human beings according to the "phallic-castrated" dichotomy and finally succeeded, but . . . at what price?

Notes

1 In German *Selbstverständlich:* "It goes without saying" but also "it is self-evident", which implies that Hans is really foolish for not having understood all by himself a situation that those around him did everything to hide from him
2 My emphasis. Did he not see her at the same time as her mother and the bloody bowls?
3 *Groß* in German can mean tall or fat.

Chapter 3

The guilt of the child's desire

Sexuality, castration and guilt

At a very early stage in his work, Freud (1909) attributed a meaning to the freedom of verbal expression and absence of guilt that can be observed in very young children when formulating their desires and phantasies in the domain of sexuality that would subsequently remain central throughout his metapsychology. This freedom can only exist prior to the expression of a threat of castration, in a space/time during which desires are not as yet sanctioned by the genital Oedipal rivalry of sexual desires. In this Garden of Eden prior to any threats and rivalry, sexuality manifests itself, therefore, without any guilt, as the notion of transgression simply does not exist.

Concerning the genesis of psychic functioning and the aetiology of its dysfunctioning in neurosis or psychotic states, all the later developments regarding the question of infantile sexuality could be considered as a decondensation of the discoveries set out in the *Three Essays on the Theory of Sexuality* (Freud, 1905).

The need to situate, within the richness of Freud's discoveries, the topography, dynamics and economy of these crucial concepts of desire and guilt requires us to define and articulate more clearly:

1 Desire and the freedom of the verbal expression of sexuality in very young children.
2 The economic status of the conscious and unconscious aspects of infantile sexual theories.
3 The differentiation between Oedipal organization and genital organization.
4 The conscious and unconscious aspects of desire and guilt in the pregenital organization.

On the first point mentioned earlier, the case of Little Hans (Freud, 1909) offers us a delightful example of the expression of desire and guilt in young children, whereas the case of the Wolf Man (Freud, 1918 [1914]) provides us with the counter-example of someone who had immobilized on a lasting basis the sexual expressions of his childhood in a painfully exaggerated sadomasochistic compulsion of disavowed desire and split-off guilt.

In the last chapter we looked at the economic status of infantile sexual theories. Freud speaks of them as if he took them for the direct expression of the child's phantasies, owing to the apparent frankness of their formulation. For my part, I think that, at a very early stage, the child only speaks the language that he hopes will be heard – we can find many examples of this in Little Hans – and that, consequently, the conscious verbalization of infantile sexual theories is a more or less sophisticated form of disguise of the expression of desire. However, even if their visible and conscious aspect which is part of verbal communication only represents the visible part of the iceberg, these theories nonetheless govern, in my view, the essential unconscious forms taken by primal phantasies. They may therefore be considered as the crucible of the different expressions of the child's desire, as found in the organization of infantile neurosis.

Both in Freud's work and thereafter, this question of the differentiation between the Oedipal and genital organizations saw developments in various directions, in particular, with the exploration by Karl Abraham (1924) of the notion of "libidinal stages" and with that of the "early Oedipus complex" posited by Melanie Klein (1932). To recapitulate briefly on the question, I would say that no serious psychoanalyst today can deny the presence of guilt in the child, well before the moment when the genital expression of his Oedipus complex becomes manifest for the outside observer. Moreover, the orientation of the aggregate of current studies in neonatology, all trends included, is to consider that a triad, not only interactive but also intrapsychic, exists in the newborn infant. If the question of the Oedipal specificity of such a triadic structure naturally remains open, this merely leads thinkers in metapsychology to dissociate even further the question of guilt from the classical description of the Oedipal organization, as described by Freud, but never to deny the early existence of this guilt.

But what is more important, in my view, is the essentially unconscious quality both of desire and guilt, from the very beginnings of psychic life. Admittedly, in order to be recognized, this quality implies the prerequisite of Freud's second conceptualization of the unconscious (Freud, 1920): the unconscious as a reservoir of phantasies, and not only as a container of the repressed. I adhere to this conceptualization all the more readily in that for me it does not imply any restriction regarding the economic and structural requirements of the drive organization at the level of the vicissitudes of its object-related and identificatory expressions.

Polymorphism and perversion: two drive vicissitudes in relation to their objects

In Freudian metapsychology there is a virtual point of departure where guilt is absent from desire. This point, which was formulated by Freud (1905) when he asserted that children are polymorphously perverse, is a good illustration of the spirit in which Freud wanted to present his discovery of infantile sexuality, attempting to conciliate the categories of classical psychopathology with the apparent freedom of expression of sexuality that he observed in young children. About seventy years after the publication of the *Three Essays*, in *The Psychoanalytic Process*, Donald Meltzer (1967), took up again, with the aim of disconnecting them, the two terms – perverse and polymorphous – contained in Freud's assertion. It was at the level of the status of the object, very different in each case, that Meltzer was to distinguish between "polymorphism" and "perversion". Following up on Freud's studies on the splitting of the ego and perversion on the one hand, and Kleinian studies on the splitting of the object and part-object relations on the other, Meltzer recalled the importance of the idealization of the bad object and, consequently, of sadomasochism, in issues of perversion, with the implications for identification that go with it. He contrasted with it the plasticity of the cathexes and identifications of polymorphism in which organized sadomasochism plays no role; on the other hand, there is a vigorous epistemophilic impulse.

It is important to note that, if such a disconnection seemed possible for Meltzer, this was because for him, after the discoveries formulated by Freud concerning Little Hans, guilt remained a concept intrinsically attached to the concept of drives, whose force and organizational originality constitute an inescapable individual factor.

If we add to that the necessity, postulated by Freud (1950 [1895]) from the "Project" onwards in various forms of an object/aim for the drive, a necessity that led him to describe the transition from need to desire, it becomes possible to consider that *there is no drive without an object and no desire without guilt.*

Deprivation and guilt

The inescapable role of object-cathexis for human development can be seen in the ordinary daily clinical practice of the psychoanalyst who systematically finds in the analysis of adult patients who suffered significant traumas in their early childhood, intense feelings of guilt for having damaged the parental objects who failed them in one way or another. The need for ego-coherence leads them to provide themselves with this kind of explanation which is intended to protect their love-objects.

Depending on the intensity and nature of the subject's drive organization and of the deprivation suffered, there will be diverse and varied drive reversals.

When object-deprivation becomes extreme, these drive reversals can no longer occur, and what we will then witness is the pure and simple extinction of the drive leading the subject to death. As evidence of this one only has to think of the edifying story of the abduction of new-born babies by Frederick II of Sicily (1194–1250) who wanted to discover the basic language of humanity. Therefore, he commanded wet-nurses to take great care of some babies but under no circumstances to utter a single word in their presence. Frederick II never discovered the secret of the basic language because all the babies died. . .

Thus it can be said that verbal contact governs in a vital way the birth of the mind of the human being, and that, in turn, its development plays a significant role in the individual's somatic survival. Now all these changes occur through the relationship with the object, which is marked by desire and guilt in both protagonists.

Primary maternal space, phallic/castrated model and identifications

Following on from the preceding discussion, and by way of transition, I would like to recall briefly that I described (Bégoin-Guignard, 1987) *the psychic space occupied in the infant by the unconscious image of the first configuration of his relationship to the world, insofar as this configuration is indispensable for psychic birth, that is for the establishment of a basic mode of functioning, as the "primary maternal space".*

This basic mode of functioning, constituted by elementary exchange mechanisms between an outside and an inside that are physically, if not psychically, delimited, may be described as an aggregate comprising:

1 Projection and introjection as mechanisms already present and functional at birth.
2 Splitting and normal projective identification as products of the first postnatal relations of identification.

I have already shown (Guignard, 1988) the importance of maternal and feminine identifications in the organization of masculine identity. These identifications imply, for the boy in the latency period, a process of mourning feminine jouissance and the capacity to give birth, in order to pave the way for a good genital cathexis of his penis at puberty. It is thanks to the psychic work required by mourning his mothers' female sexual organs that the little boy will identify with her feminine and maternal aspects. The phallic/castrated model is therefore a convenient sexual theory erected as a reaction formation with the aim of avoiding this work of mourning.

As for the little girl, it is in the delay of this period of latency linked to mourning the sexual organ that she does not have that the essential aspects of her masculine and paternal identifications will be formed. Her reaction formation will consist in a negation of the phallic/castrated model – which amounts to its affirmation – in the form of so-called "tomboy" behaviour.

Furthermore, she will compete with the feminine and maternal aspects of her mother out of what is often an envious desire to possess the contents of the mother's body, a desire whose misery will assume various forms ranging from hypochondria to the most severe somatizations.

Primary feminine space, lack, introjective identification and psychic bisexuality

Following on from the "primary maternal" space, a second psychic space is organized and I have chosen to call it the "primary feminine" space in tribute to the importance, for my considerations, of the discovery by Melanie Klein (1932) of the "primary feminine phase". Common to the children of both sexes, this relational and identificatory configuration which appears between the ages of 4 and 6 months results from the conjunction of two trends:

1 An intensification of oral sadism that is linked to teething and organizes phantasies related to weaning;
2 The appearance of a specific desire for the father's penis through identification with the mother's desire for it.

For Klein, this configuration has two logical consequences: an upsurge of capacities for introjection at the level of development and, from a psychopathological point of view, this configuration is described as a fixation-point for male homosexuality.

Thus, the primary feminine space may be defined as the psychic space occupied, in the infant, by the unconscious image of the configuration corresponding to the de-idealization of the mother/baby pair, the end of the honeymoon period, of the mother's normal state of illness – which, even if normal, is nonetheless an illness. The parents' life as a couple and family life reclaim their rights just at the point when the infant is increasingly ready to effect displacements of cathexes. I therefore consider the primary feminine space as the psychic space that develops in connection with the first triangulation observable in the human being. It is the first space of absence, of the negative, of the mutual "letting go" in the mother/baby dyad and, consequently, of any potentiality of the processes of mourning.

The economic equilibrium of psychic bisexuality in connection with the biological sex of the individual will depend on this space being well established.

In terms of the description of psychic functioning, the constitution of this new field of cathexis will involve a complexification and reorganization of the infant's mode of relating, in both its narcissistic and object-related aspects. Indeed, he will be able to organize increasingly complex relations between the primary maternal field and the primary feminine field. Likewise, the organization of his identifications will draw more significantly on his mechanisms of introjection, leading to an increase in introjective identifications. In my view, the latter can be quite easily defined with reference to the model of culture, of which it is said that "it is what is left when we have forgotten everything". Now I consider that the nucleus of the ego is constituted, precisely, by introjective identifications and that consequently its vicissitudes are linked to those of the feminine.

Desire, reality and guilt in children's play

As a result, all human, intrapsychic, interpersonal and group experiences, all the scenarios of learning in the broad sense of the term, will be woven in the interaction of these two spaces, of these two modes of object-relating and identification that are characteristic of the primary maternal and primary feminine spaces. It is from this process of weaving that the space for playing, which Edouard Clarapède (1905) said was the work of the child, emerges. Play – we only need to think of Freud's (1920) wooden-reel game and Winnicott's (1965) spatula game – also interests and raises questions for psychoanalysis, and the child analyst knows very well that it is a royal road leading to the child's phantasy life which is analogous (but not identical) to that of the dream narrative (but not the dream) for the adult's phantasy life.

Klein (1923, 1926, 1929) pursued very boldly – to great lengths – the analysis of play and the theoretical hypotheses derived from it. For her, play enables the child to expel the most guilt-inducing aspects of his parental superego. Admittedly, this expulsion is only temporary and must be worked on in the context of the transference relationship, precisely from the angle of the unconscious guilt of the ego in relation to its most imposing internal object: the superego.

Inhibition is the most frequent pathology in the organization of the psychic space of play. A child that does not play becomes, as a result, a child who falls ill on account of the unconscious guilt of his desire and of his rejection of reality, through what is called – somewhat mechanically – his intolerance of frustration. In analysis, this intolerance varies considerably from one patient to another, whether adult or child. In spite of all the aetiological hypotheses that have been advanced on this subject, it is a factor that often resists analytic techniques and which unfailingly induces a negative transference, or a negative therapeutic reaction.

The analyst's margin for manoeuvre is then very narrow, ranging from silence that may be experienced as cruel and interpretations that may be more of a hindrance than a help. Certainly, the analyst is aware of the example of Klein who, in such circumstances, was able to overcome the child's inhibition by interpreting his fear of the possibility of retaliation in connection with his sadistic impulses; but the child in question is different and the analyst is not Klein. A little imagination, a great deal of patience and, above all, sensitivity and tact, often lead the child to use, or to discover, a space for playing.

However, autistic children, psychotic children and certain borderline children do not have a sufficient degree of inner freedom to develop a playful relationship with others – in short, they are unable either to engage in *play* or to take part in *games* – according to Winnicott's terminology. Others, who have been able to play in a meaningful and fruitful way, stop playing one day, either gradually or all of a sudden, because they are so bogged down in a mode of unconscious functioning in which phantasy seems to be experienced as dangerously externalized, threatening as if it were real, in the form of a symbolic equation. As I have tried to show (Guignard, 1994a), this de-symbolization of the session material is the mark of the effects of a blind spot in the countertransference.

Another pathology of play is stereotypy. Klein comes to our help here once again, when she recommends remaining attentive to the slightest variations that occur between two versions of the same game. Here, too, it is important to explore our countertransference, particularly in the domain of our conflict between cathecting what is the same and what is different. It may be that we will discover our own unconscious eroticization at work in the attempt to preserve obsessionally *what is the same* even though, at a conscious level, it exasperates us.

Depressive guilt and Oedipal desire

Klein's observation that the early appearance of genital impulses plays an important role in psychic organization is of great importance in understanding the economy of the drives, relationships and identifications in a nascent state. This implies that the early advent of genital impulses favours the emergence of Oedipal preforms of desire and guilt. It is my contention that the Kleinian concept of the "central depressive position" is precisely *the direct metapsychological expression of the mise en abyme of this desire and guilt.*

The consequences of this configuration essentially concern the value and significance to be given to the movements of individuation of the infant. The metapsychological perspective that I am elaborating leads to observing the way in which these movements organize relations between the elements of the ego and the elements of its introjected objects. It will be recalled that, for Freud, the very first of these objects is in the order of the superego, which Klein (1928; 1933; 1945) accepted and developed with her concept of "early superego".

It is therefore essential for the practising psychoanalyst to focus his research on the question of desire and guilt, which, at the same time, become very early organizers. Admittedly, the obligation to take them into account means that we forfeit once again the myth of the "green paradise of childhood loves". On the other hand, we will gain the possibility of paying closer attention to, and of seeking a more precise meaning for, the events – somatic, familial and psychic – that may have occurred in the very first months of life, forming for the subject a traumatic point with prolonged effects.

Guilt and the thirst for knowledge

In the last chapter, we saw the emerging curiosity of Little Hans the investigator. Further on, we will see the imaginary dialogue between Leonardo and Freud on the subject of the thirst for knowledge and love. It is worth pointing out here that, following in Freud's footsteps, Klein (1930; 1931) integrates the epistemophilic impulse with her work as a whole. As for Bion (1965), he organizes his entire psychoanalytic theory of thinking around a drive tripod[1] that attributes as much importance to the thirst for knowledge (+K) as to love (+L) and to hate (+H), as well as to their respective negative forms (-K), (-L) and (-H), which constitute what I refer to as their entropic value.

In child psychopathology, we are confronted on a daily basis with the problem of -K. Anyone who has tried to work in psychoanalytic psychotherapy with children presenting a developmental deficit, whether harmonious or disharmonious, knows how much unconscious guilt linked to the thirst for knowledge is at its height in this kind of psychic organization. We should therefore be able to approach this kind of problem from three complementary angles:

1 The guilt linked to the thirst for knowledge about the content of the primal phantasies: seduction, castration, primal scene, and scene of origins.
2 The guilt linked to the wish to penetrate the object who is supposed to know, in order to extract this knowledge from him more or less violently.
3 The guilt linked to the processes of introjective identification which alone permit the subject to appropriate this knowledge, at the price

of moving away from the fusional mode of relating with the primary objects.

The multidisciplinary research studies that I conducted (Guignard et al. 1965; Guignard et al. 1972; Guignard,1972) for ten years at the instigation of Julian de Ajuriaguerra, confirmed the major importance of taking into account these dynamic factors of personality for the success of re-educational approaches to all "dys" disorders: dyspraxias, dysphasias, dyslexias, etc.

Note

1 I am intentionally retaining Bion's terms in English (L, K, H), as I share his concern to get rid of as many "saturated" conceptual terms as possible, which are much too polysemic as a result to be precise and scientifically useful. Notably, here, he uses *knowledge* to refer to the "thirst for knowledge" in the sense of the epistemophilic impulse, and not to "knowledge" as a philosophical category.

Chapter 4

The sources of projective identification

When Klein (1945) described the archaic aspects of the Oedipus complex and, in so doing, discovered that at these levels the mind functions in a different way than in neurotic functioning, as observed by Freud, the term that she came upon to describe this archaic mode of functioning was that of "psychotic". She never reneged on this term, which was subsequently taken up by all Kleinian and post-Kleinian authors, and particularly by Bion. It would be problematic and unscientific not to try to understand what she meant by it, and furthermore it would entail splitting off and denying the importance of her discoveries for psychoanalytic thought.

The two axes of this research can be found in "Notes on some schizoid mechanisms' (Klein, 1946) with, on the one hand, the extension of the Freudian concept of splitting and, on the other, the introduction of the concept of projective identification.

In order to explore identifications that Freud (1917a [1915]) had identified as narcissistic, Klein revisits, with the aim of examining and extending it to the object, the concept of the splitting of the ego (Freud, 1940[1938)]) as a defensive process connected with perversion. The subject's statement "I know, but all the same", led her to grasp the whole difficulty of the boundaries between external reality and psychic reality, and she understood that the narcissistic fantasy is a fantasy of gaining power over all or part of an object in external reality. The subject projects his omnipotence into it and can henceforth identify with it in a very particular way that enables him to circumvent the painful work of mourning and renunciation required by the post-Oedipal introjective identifications described by Freud.

She therefore discovered that the object is also split – and not only the ego – and thereby opened up the whole field of exploration of part-object relations. Consequently, the primary narcissistic state could no longer be considered as an objectless state, since each split-off part of the ego can, potentially, be combined with each split-off part of the object, external or internal. Freud (1921) had already noted that narcissistic identifications are generally formed on the basis of a single detail perceived in the person who is the object of the identification. Seen through the projective glasses of a part of the ego, a part of the real object becomes simultaneously an external object of desire and an internal object of identification, in the sense of Fontaine's fable in which the jay is decked in the peacock's feathers. The statement "I desire the object" corresponds exactly to the statement "I am the desirable object". There are therefore two residues: the residue of the ego and the residue of the person as an object of desire and an object of projective identification. Both of these residues will be subject to denial, which justifies the description "schizoid" applied to these mechanisms by Klein. Thus, the remarkably efficient combination of splitting, denial and projective identification will guarantee the formidably autarkic character of the narcissistic state that Freud had found so striking.

And yet, in the movement that drove her once again – following Freud's example, moreover, to explore pathology, Klein was not afraid to assert that these schizoid mechanisms are constitutive of normal development. The descriptions that she gives of the struggle of the ego, splitting itself with the aim of cathecting objects that are themselves split by it, offended the feelings of many readers who had forgotten that it was Freud himself who had destroyed the myth of the monism of the personality, initially by discovering the existence of the unconscious, and then by describing the ego and its relations with its most important internal object, the superego.

With this new combination, the model of the world of psychic relations took on an unforeseen spatial complexity: the inside and outside of the internal psychic world – the *Self* of Anglo-Saxon authors –, of the internal objects within the Self, of the ego and of external objects would all become part of a moving and complicated interplay of relations and identifications with each other, in totality or in part, through the perpetual movement of projection/introjection that I like to describe as "psychic respiration".

The extreme complexity of psychic life does not, however, reside only in this plurality of spaces and objects, or even in the combination of this plurality with the disparity between the force and respective phases of projection and introjection. This complexity lies specifically in the plurality of meanings conveyed by each of the projective and introjective drive movements towards each of these spaces of the Self and of the external world. For none of these meanings is unequivocal. But none is equivocal either, in the sense in which Freud (1940 [1938)]) understood it in the "Splitting of the ego in the process of defence". At any rate, they can only become equivocal at a very sophisticated conscious level – "I know, but all the same" – while at the unconscious level each of these meanings has the imperious concreteness of fantasy, of an emotion that has barely emerged from raw sensory data, an infra symbolic protothought, in the kingdom of primary processes and thing-presentations. This is why the "interpretation of psychic reality" (Begoin, 1982) is comprised of a plurality of levels

of experience among which the analyst will have to choose, guided by the thread of the transference and his countertransference insight.

Developments and evaluations of the concept

In Chapter 2, I tried to show how, with his theory of thinking, Bion offered a crucial extension of the concept of projective identification by treating it as the normal function of intersubjective communication; moreover, he considered that it was absolutely indispensable for the establishment of psychic life in the infant.

Meltzer (1978), for his part, criticized the term projective identification in its Kleinian sense and, had it not been for the force of custom, would have preferred the term "intrusive identification". He also contributed (Meltzer, 1983) to describing the broad spectrum covered by this concept today by proposing a classification of the psychopathology in the light of the various modes of projective identification and of the various spaces that it occupies in psychic reality. According to him, certain pathological forms involve more particularly the identificatory aspect of projective identification, that is, the pathology of the aspect of the immediate appropriation of the qualities of the object. The most obvious example of this is hysterical conversion. The identificatory aspect is equally in the foreground in manic-depressive psychosis, in states of pseudo-maturity (see further on), and in severe hypochondria, studied brilliantly by Herbert Rosenfeld (1965). In this last condition, the fantasy of having been unjustly deprived of a nourishing and helpful object leads the subject to seek aid from the external object aid. He will then secretly denigrate this aid and repeatedly render it ineffective owing to the intensity of his affects of envy and desires for revenge against an object who ought to lead him to abandon his omnipotence insofar as he depends on him.

The hypochondriac, who identifies projectively with the very object whom he secretly intrudes upon, presents a polymorphism of his parasitic projections. This does not, however, diminish the potential malignity of his pathology, ranging from hysteria to psychosomatic illness – hence the sense of triumph of hypochondriacs when they succumb to a confirmed illness. Meltzer (1978) sees this occurrence of a somatic illness as the concretization of the fantasy of a paranoid object, produced by the alliance of a bad internal object with a hateful part of the ego.

In what he calls "somatic delusion", the interpretative delusion is organized more specifically around the cunning ploy of the parasitic part of the subject. The projective identification into an external object inhabited by this predatory guest is potentialized by powerful splitting aimed at better concealing the ascendancy over the object. It is not uncommon, in the course of an analysis, to discover an encysted delusion which it is difficult to know what to do with. Somatic delusion is a particularly difficult variant of it to detect, and also very tricky to handle due to the very precarious state of the function of symbolization in such patients at high risk of somatization.

For the analyst, the risk lies in the intensity of the defences that he will tend to set up in his countertransference with a view to protecting himself against the latent envy of the patient, who will continually attack the gains of the analytic work – in particular the reestablishment of splitting that is appropriate for the operation of thought and the attribution of judgement – in order to sow confusion in the analytic space. If the analyst is unable to enter into contact with this state of confusion, he will make serious errors of appreciation as to the nature and quality of the transference objects that he represents for his patient. The more the analytic work is impeded by the pathology of the patient's processes of splitting, the greater the temptation will be for the psychoanalyst to attribute a symbolic meaning to the manifest content of the dreams and associations of such a patient. The patient will therefore always be able to make us take pigs' ears for silk purses and delusional anti-thinking for fantasies.

Other pathological forms involve more particularly the projective aspect of projective identification, that is, the state of the object's internal world as fantasized, at least, by the subject. It is clearly the domain of the phobias that is concerned, and in particular the nature and quality of the atmosphere that reigns in the object – a prototypical feature of claustrophobia. Another aspect of this projective aspect of projective identification can be observed in certain confusional psychotic states, particularly in adolescence.

In the "interpretative syndrome", there is clearly a pathology of the projective aspect of projective identification, since the patient is convinced that he knows what the other person thinks. Such patients may appear, at first sight, to be gifted with remarkable insight concerning the disorders for which they are seeking treatment. They give so much meaning to the material they bring that they could, it seems, do their analysis by themselves. Moreover, they are not the only objects of their thoughtful remarks. Gradually, their analyst notices that such patients conduct themselves with him like *mediums* and are able to tell him so many pertinent – and irrelevant – things about himself that it wouldn't take much for him to be ready to pay them. Everything would be fine in the best of all possible worlds if, one way or another, the analyst were not tempted, in spite of everything, to intervene by proposing, in his turn, an interpretation. The metamorphosis is then spectacular: he finds himself in front of a concrete wall erected by a patient who is ready to employ any delusional formations, even murderous or suicidal, to avoid living within his own psychic territory.

If, after a more or less lengthy period of repetition, it is relatively easy for the experienced analyst to recover his capacity for thinking with such delusional patients, it proves trickier when he is dealing with a borderline patient who uses normal projective identification, albeit too intensely. This is because the significant figures in his early environment had little or no capacity for thinking and, in any case, never made such capacities available to the patient in a relationship of intimacy. Deprived of a reliable container to help them cope with their problem of object-loss, they use their projective identification for the purposes of understanding those who do not take the trouble to understand them. They thus acquire a pseudo-maturity, like the 10-year-old child who, when presenting himself to me for the first time, said to me very simply: "I'm my mother's mother". Unfortunately, this was perfectly exact from the point of view of the capacities that this child had to use projection to identify with his mother's conflicts and to contain them; but he accomplished this immense psychic work at the price of tragic distress and immaturity regarding his own development and capacities for autonomy. There is a clear convergence here with Winnicott's concept of the "false-self". The countertransference trap that we offer such patients is that of mutual projective identification at the level of our own Infantile, thereby taking the risk of functioning in a vacuum like two children equally gifted for interpretation.

The range of the processes of projective identification

Are we in a position, at this point in our reflection, to determine whether the process of projective identification as such is of a psychotic nature or not?

My clinical practice suggests that it is as much a matter of universal and daily usage as the Oedipal configuration. When it is operative in the capacity for reverie characteristic of the mother and the psychoanalyst, it can be considered as one of the offshoots of the Oedipal issues of the parents.

On the contrary, just as projective identification can be constitutive of meaning, so can it be constitutive of non-meaning each time it is used defensively against castration or annihilation anxieties that are too overwhelming. The more the ego is weak and the sense of identity uncertain, the more threatening these anxieties are. That is why projective identification will be used all the more massively, intrusively or pathologically when the subject is fragile, in whatever respect that may be. A particular inner intolerance for frustration or a particularly and repeatedly frustrating external situation (specifically, the deafness of the immediate environment to the subject's psychic life), can even result in projective identification becoming caught up in a vicious circle of repetition compulsion, potentialized by the compelling necessity to resort to multiple splitting to avoid breakdown.

Sometimes a breakdown happens. Psychotic confusion then sets in, the processes of splitting and projective identification will function aberrantly in a world whose axes of reference – good/bad, nourishing relationship/sexual relationship, self/others, masculine/feminine, adult/child – will be totally distorted.

Klein's (1946) *key* description of the mechanisms of splitting, denial, idealization and projective identification as the very first mechanisms of defence, and as constituent elements of primary relationships and primary identifications, retains all its worth, provided that two clarifications are added:

1 No psychic life can emerge without the help of the psychic life of another human being who uses their normal processes of projective identification for the purpose of "dreaming" the psychic existence of the newborn baby.
2 These mechanisms of splitting and projective identification, the constituent elements of the paranoid-schizoid position (Klein, 1946), must be understood as being the most frequent but not the only defensive complex that is used at an early stage against suffering inherent to the central depressive position, that is to say to what I would call the long march towards elaborating the loss of the object. The whole pathology of narcissism may be considered as an omnipotent (Rosenfeld, 1987) use of projective identification as a defence against the loss of the object, experienced as a loss of the Self. Klein (1940) considered the suffering that goes with the elaboration of the depressive position as the worst that the human being has to endure in order to gain access to his true identity through the advent of the function of symbolization.

In any case, each one of us will function throughout life with the help of the processes of projective identification. Projective identification is a spontaneous and immediate response to the stimuli coming from the outside or the inside, and a permanent attempt to give a first level of meaning to the relationships with others and with our internal objects. It is the mechanism through which desire – one's own and that of the other – can pass, as many symbolic forms of behaviour show: from the handshake to the peace pipe, including the kiss and greetings cards, the human being will always seek in one way or another to "figure out" his neighbour by means of a projective identification with the desire of the other.

Furthermore, projective identification, – normal, it is to be hoped – is the psychoanalyst's working instrument par excellence. It enables him to get in contact with a mind whose characteristics may be very different from his own, which is unknown but not completely foreign because it is human, and which formulates a desire concerning him. Only projective identification can help him to take the measure of this desire and to explore its nature; whereupon, he will have to introject and digest this emotional experience so that the analytic process can get underway.

Along the path of the countertransference we meet many stumbling blocks, the most important of which will not only stem from our patients. Among those that concern us, I would like to note in particular:

1 The need to detect the defensive pole of our countertransference projective identification – on this subject see the remarkable contributions of León Grinberg (1962; 2018) on projective counter-identification.
2 The need to be able to use our processes of projective identification for the purpose of experiencing the extremely violent and often overwhelming affects projected into us by our analysands, such as sexual excitation, hate, terrorism, despair, murderous and suicidal wishes, but also scorn, arrogance, mania, prejudices of all kinds, narcissistic self-satisfaction, the force of habit and, last but not least, mental confusion and the sense of absolute foolishness when faced with the material that is presented to us in the session.

The psychoanalyst's projective identification is a doubled-edged sword: without it, we are simply chatting with our patients *on the subject* of psychoanalysis and we are not functioning as psychoanalysts, that is, at the level of affects and representations. With it, we constantly run the risk of falling into mutual projection in which the treatment will get bogged down, and as a result the analytic process will come undone.

Obviously, the most that we can hope for, both for our analysands and for ourselves, is to plunge into it with the aim of touching the bottom of emotional experience, while emerging from it again through the work of elaborating our thought-processes, analogous to the dream-work. It goes without saying that we will never get to the bottom of things, but this determination to try, at least, to do so seems to me to be commensurate with our presumption – an exorbitant one, when all is said and done – of offering another human being our help in the form of interpreting his transferential relationship with us.

To leave this place of practice and its limits is to succumb to omnipotence and repetition compulsion, the gates of entry to the hell of the psychotic interpretation of the world.

Chapter 5

The depressive position and the Oedipus complex

Although in the second part of her work, Melanie Klein gave pride of place to the genetic sense of the concept of the "depressive position", it would be a serious distortion of the history of psychoanalytic concepts to overlook the very first description of this notion. Indeed, in her first contributions, Klein (1921) established the depressive position as the central position, the key position in the advent of psychic life, individuation and symbolization. Since the other positions are set up by an embryonic ego as defensive measures against the psychic suffering linked to the reality principle that determines the depressive position, it is the paranoid-schizoid position that constitutes the defensive position, *prima inter pares*, owing to the immediate efficacy of its mode of regressive organization to a world where everything is split and described in Manichean fashion, including the Self and its objects of cathexis. Hence Bion's (1965) conceptualization: PS ↔ D, which establishes a new link between metapsychology and philosophy by insisting on the dynamic, oscillatory and regulating character in daily life of these two poles of the basic psychic organization.

It was Klein (1928) who described the early structures of the Oedipal configuration. She identifies its point of departure immediately after the constitution of the depressive position, towards the middle of the first year of life. The inevitable consequence of the differentiation between self and others is merely the discovery of the third element.

Rather than repudiating this contribution of clinical practice to theory, or to avoid it by means of subtle distinctions between the triangles that are supposedly Oedipal and those that are not, it seems more fruitful to me to examine the way in which the combined interplay of the two parameters PS ↔ D and the early Oedipus complex challenges today our classical conception of the "Oedipus complex at the age of 3", and therefore, our materials of reconstruction in analysis. I have chosen to examine three of these junction points:

1 The first concerns the usefulness of a conceptualization in terms of part-objects for understanding and interpreting defences against the depressive position and Oedipal conflicts.

2 The second concerns the impact of post-Freudian contributions on the parameters of the technique of interpretation throughout a psychoanalyst's life, parameters that are real or fantasized by the psychoanalytic community to which he belongs.
3 The third concerns the importance and nature of the processes of identification, both in the advent of interpretation in the psychoanalyst and in the way in which the analysand receives it.

Part-objects and red thread

I am inclined to think that the reality of the movements of affects can never be conceptualized adequately if we use the monistic model of a single intrapsychic conflictual knot. The unity of the patient's ego, a unity in the name of which this monistic conceptualization is recommended to analysts as a technical tool, would, on the contrary, be much weakened and impoverished by an analytic technique that operated on the basis of such a simplification of unconscious processes. Trying to gather all the emotional impulses around a red thread – that is to say, tracing all the difficulties of being a patient back to a single organizing knot of complexes – amounts to suggesting to a sailor that he should only use one rope to steer his boat, which, even for the British navy, raises some difficulties in the case of a gale. But above all, it radically eliminates any possibility of unfurling the sails and, *mutatis mutandis*, any possibility of developing other parts of the ego and internal objects, which are thus split-off and rejected, by the analyst himself, outside the transference relationship. Here we are touching on the limits and dangers of metaphorization, and I do not doubt that Freud, in speaking of the red thread, had in mind the need for a plurality of threads. It is in the transmission of the theory of the technique that the evocative richness of metaphors is lost and that they regress to a level of symbolic equations.

On the other hand, the interest of a conceptualization in terms of part-object relations and identifications with part-objects goes well beyond a possible genetic point of view. This way of describing the intrapsychic movements established by the different aspects of the ego with the different aspects of its cathected objects is essential, in my view, when trying to form a picture of the abundance and complexity of an individual's mode of psychic functioning, whether adult or child, neurotic or psychotic, in relation to the continuous emergence of symbolizing activity.

If we keep in mind Freud's discoveries, it is clear that the mode of relating in terms of part-objects constitutes the mode of expression par excellence of the unconscious. This description of the unconscious functioning of the subject/object relationship falls within exactly the same perspective as Freud's (1900) description of the functioning of dream-thoughts, on the one hand, and of thing-presentations on the other. This mode of part-object relating can therefore be observed particularly, albeit indirectly, in the dream narrative, but also – and this is crucial – in any expression of unconscious transference.

Thus, although the discovery of otherness implies by the same token the notion of a third element, it would be very naïve to think that this discovery permanently and wholly influences the subject's psychic organization. Ultimately, it would be to deny the existence of the unconscious or, at least, the struggle for influence of its logic over the territories won over by conscious logic. Furthermore, the proper development of the processes of displacement will give rise to a multitude of situations in which otherness and triangulation can come into play, making it necessary to find models of thought that are operational. Admittedly, the drastic solution that is only too familiar of making a deliberate equation between the pregenital and pre-Oedipal registers in order to apply one and the same relational schema to both boils down to throwing the baby out with the bath water. However, a valid alternative still has to be found.

The idea that the entirety of the Other and the totality of the triangular Oedipal combinations in the relationship to it might only constitute an asymptote for the human mind subject, as it is, to a double structural and temporal constraint, allows the analyst to consider his work with more modesty, but obliges him, at the same time, to be very attentive to the ideational formations that punctuate the analytic relationship. Indeed, each of them offers a point of view concerning one of the existing links between one of the aspects of the subject and one of the aspects of one of his internal objects. The interest of these points of view is that each of them contains a virtual pivotal point that the psychoanalyst can try to mobilize.

A pivotal point, that is, between a Manichean paranoid-schizoid vision of the world that is omnipotent and illusorily fusional, on the one hand, and a depressive and Oedipal vision on the other; between a narcissistic state of subject/object bemusement and an area of solitude and play that creates sufficient distance between the subject and the object so that a compromise is found that is necessary for discovering and accepting the existence of an unknown part in each of them. For all this to occur, it is necessary to have quite a precise view of the nature and quality of the part-object and of the part of the Self that constitute the protagonists of this mini-scene – mini, but potentially capable of invading all the psychic space – and to succeed in interpreting adequately the transference version of it.

Theoretical contributions and technical parameters

Every psychoanalyst has fantasies about how his colleagues work. These fantasies reflect first and foremost his ambivalence about aspects of the theoretical corpus with which he is not very familiar. Now these fantasies have an undeniably obscuring effect on his listening to the work of other analysts. However, the evolution "in waves" of the technique of interpretation can be observed, both that which that claims to be strictly Freudian and that which purports to be enriched by the contributions of other authors. In fact, within each analytic group, and each analyst, there are varying degrees of investment in the theoretical and technical parameters of the science and art of psychoanalysis, variations that are responsible for a significant portion of the unconscious choice of the parameters of interpretation. Another factor of variation in the technique of interpretation – and not the least – lies in the analyst's personal development. Finally, the style of interpretation varies and evolves with each patient to the extent that the latter's inner discourse – and not only his narrative language – linked to his infantile history, manifests itself increasingly.

For my part, I would like to highlight the advantage presented, for the analyst's thinking in session, by the *multi-dimensional* vision to which he will have access in approaching the various landscapes of the analysand's internal psychic life. Now I think it is easier to acquire this multidimensional approach without any depersonalizing effects if the analyst is able to recognize that in every neurotic patient there are conflicts inherent to the ego between the unifying tendencies and the partializing tendencies which favour splitting or fragmentation. To Freud's description of the pathological splitting of the ego in the pervert, Klein added more detailed clinical material that showed the frequency, extent and variations of the intensity and quality of the processes of splitting of the ego and of cathected objects as a mode of functioning underlying and concurrent with repression. To this I would like to add the iconographic richness the analyst derives from studying the unconscious phantasies corresponding to the relations established by these different parts of the ego with its various objects, internal and external. This richness was evoked by Freud (1923a) when he describes the ego as first and foremost a body ego, and then developed by Klein when she describes part-object relations as bringing into play the different parts of the subject's body and of his internalized parents.

Finally, I will mention the importance of the *key* description of the mode of psychic functioning of these transactions between the different parts of the ego with the different parts of its objects. This description that Freud gave in his conceptualization of the *Pcs.* in his metapsychological papers of 1915–1917, was to acquire a new amplitude and functionality when Bion elaborated his theory of thinking in order to describe the analytic relational situation. Bion characterized the latter as a "container/contained" relationship, whose signifiers are the signs: ♂♀. In this relational situation, the analyst uses his α function – in other words, his normal projective identification – to contain the more or less intrusive, or even frankly pathological, projective identifications of the patient, with the aim of promoting their development and transformation into normal projective identifications that can be used for the activity of symbolization characteristic of the activity of thinking.

Interpretation and identifications

I will begin with Bion's description of the beginning of the process of projective identification, whether normal or pathological:

> If mother and child [*mutatis mutandis*, analyst and patient] are adjusted to each other, projective identification plays a role in the management through the operation of a rudimentary and fragile reality sense; usually an omnipotent phantasy, it operates realistically. *This I am inclined to believe, is its normal condition*. . . . As a realistic activity it shows itself as behaviour reasonably calculated to *arouse in the mother feelings of which the infant wishes to be rid*. . . . If the mother cannot tolerate these projections, the infant is reduced to continued projective identification carried out with increasing force and frequency.
>
> (Bion, 1961, pp. 114–115, my emphasis)

The conceptual tool of projective identification supplements, as a term of comparison, the classical model of post-Oedipal introjective identifications described by Freud, that is, introjections that mark the identificatory predominance of the genital organization over pregenital organizations. This enables us to redistribute the identificatory impulses of our analysands according to these two major categories. Now this comparison helps us to see that in the "normal" subject, and in our Western civilizations at least, the proportion of real introjective identifications remains in fact quite low during the whole period of latency, and even during the first part of adolescence.

It may therefore be interesting, with any given patient, to use as diagnostic criteria the evaluation of the respective portion of his projective and introjective identifications, but also the appreciation of the quality – normal, intrusive or pathological – of his projective identifications at the beginning, during, and at the end of the analytic treatment. This makes it possible to evaluate the risks of an eroticized transference, of negativity and the possibility of negative therapeutic reaction, as well as the nature of the dangers of acting out and somatization.

This hypothesis is not without implications for the question of interpretations. Indeed, considered from the angle of identifications, almost all the effects of interpretation in analysis can be observed and described at the level of projective identifications. To paraphrase Freud, they are the visible part of the iceberg of identifications, while it is much more difficult to evaluate the changes that have occurred at the level of introjective identifications. However, the metaphor should be reversed concerning the proportions, and I would venture to say that in every human being nine-tenths of identifications are projective and one-tenth introjective. I would add the further observation, shared by Melzer, that the majority of the introjective identifications arising in an analytic treatment only begin to manifest themselves at its very end and even, generally speaking, after it has ended. Sometimes, therefore, there is a need for post-analytic work aimed at discovering with the patient the aspects of himself that are still in a relationship of projective identification with his analyst, and why – unless, that is, the quality of his projective identifications has not been sufficiently modified and it is necessary to envisage a new analytic adventure. As long as the quality of the analysand's projective identifications remains unsatisfactory, we can be certain that his relations to the present object as well as to the absent object have not been worked-through sufficiently, whether it is a case of Oedipal objects or of the primary object of cathexis. In these circumstances, there will be even less chance of transforming projective identifications into introjective identifications. In their place, false analytic vocations will flourish and we will see stereotyped imitations of the analyst's style, a voyeuristic fixation on the latter's deeds and gestures. In short, the true self will be parasited by the false-self. There is a big risk, as we know, that this will end in a serious depressive crisis, whose only outcome will consist in a reversal of love into hate, ranging from adhesion to the analytic way of thinking to an iconoclastic rebellion of the parental objects narcissistically cathected in the person of the analyst. Sometimes it is possible to see in this a reactivation of the means used by the patient in his past to try to reach, against all odds, an elusive parental object. Patients who have suffered significant traumas in their early childhood or adolescence are familiar with this, and very often they are the ones who confront us with our own technical errors, in particular the difficulty of being able to distinguish between a signal of psychic distress and a reaction of aggressive or sadistic intrusiveness.

Chapter 6

A stroll in the preconscious*

The drives and their objects

Agreeing to contribute to the task of revising metapsychological concepts is, it seems to me, rather like accepting an invitation to the perpetual tea-party of the March Hare in *Alice in Wonderland* by Lewis Carroll (1869): when a new guest arrives, everybody shifts up by one place and only the newcomer will have a clean tea cup – at least, as long as there is unused crockery. This means that, in my opinion, we have every chance – minus one, reserved for the genius of Freud – of discovering that our tea cup is only a remake of that of our neighbours, in terms not only of the contents but also of the container. Our only chance, after all, is to make the best use of the ingredients that our predecessors have left us and to try, by adding our own, to make in turn a drinkable beverage in two respects: scientifically digestible because it obeys the reality principle, and qualitatively pleasant – *plaisirable* would be the appropriate term if it existed in English – in order to mark the pleasure principle. A painful danger awaits us however: if our way of dreaming metapsychology annoyed the other guests too much, we could well suffer the fate of the Dormouse, which was, it will be remembered, brutally repressed and driven back into the teapot of the unconscious, where he is now stewing without disturbing anyone.

But it is to Alice-the-Ego that it falls, as usual, to foresee the worst danger: what will happen when the first of the guests has gone right round the table? As we know, she is rebuffed for the insolence of her question, and her dream takes on a new course. It might nevertheless be interesting if every psychoanalyst were to pursue his dream in search of a solution to this problem. In fact, eighty years ago, our first guest, Freud, left the immense table he had set for us without having been round it. Other guests, more or less brilliant, followed him, starting with Karl Abraham and Sándor Ferenczi. And our problem now is to know what to do while waiting to suffer the common fate. Certainly, the simplest solution, apparently – but only apparently – might be to bring one's own personal cup. In fact, this situation in external reality obviously has its internal counterpart, and we know of guests, such as Karl Gustav Jung or Alfred Adler, who did not wait to die before leaving the Freudian table. Among those who stayed, few brought with them a cup that was both new and in harmony with the Freudian corpus, by which I mean, adequate to contain the authentic psychoanalytic beverage: Klein declared her loyalty and was rejected into the outer darkness; Winnicott was viewed in the eyes of certain eminent French colleagues as a "Scottish nanny"; and Bion had to leave the old continent to be recognized a posteriori. Admittedly, we sometimes wash our dirty dishes in private – the conference of the British Society on Child Analysis,[1] centred on Anna Freud and Melanie Klein, remains the prototypical model of a situation which, since then and elsewhere, has featured much more vile quarrels. In fact, we sometimes break analytical dishes; badly contained in chipped containers, and even broken into a thousand pieces, the Freudian beverage is dispersed and ends up being lost. For those of us who live within what Bion called the Establishment, the most common danger is also the most insidious, namely, refusing to acknowledge that the *tour de table* has been completed, and so starting it all over again in denial of a compulsion to repeat that is all the deadlier because it claims to be conservative. Indeed, the primary role of the analytic group is to be the guardian of Freudian orthodoxy, that is to say of a certain number of invariants. However, since the object of this analytical science is a living object, these invariants will not only be witnesses to permanence, but also to transformation – Bion again. This means that the action of the death drive must not escape the conceptual re-examination that we will carry out for the sake of orthodoxy. Certainly, there are human beings whose dimensions of genius do not allow for mourning, in the sense of a sufficiently stable work of introjective identification. Freud is, of course, one of those whose lively and revolutionary thought will never cease to disturb us. It will depend, however, on the nature and qualities of our processes of mourning and introjection of the thought-processes of our elders whether or not we have enough security and freedom in our internal relationships with them to develop some foresight about our commensal position and, possibly, about the situation of the table of our psychoanalytic community.

Need I say that the background of my tea cup consists, for the present work, in a constant re-reading of the writings of Freud, in particular – but not only – on metapsychology? Among the innumerable vectors suggested by this re-reading, I was tempted to approach here the question of the preconscious as a geometrical space where two vectors meet: the drives and their objects on the one hand, and the vicissitudes of the container/contained relationship on the other hand.

In "A note on the unconscious in psychoanalysis", Freud (1912) approaches with great caution the question of the preconscious, using it in its adjectival form and granting it a very vague status. He says for example that "the distinction between foreconscious and unconscious activities is not a primary one, but comes to be established after repulsion has sprung up" (p. 264), but also that:

> The latent thoughts of the dream differ in no respect from the products of our regular conscious activity; they deserve the name of foreconscious thoughts and may indeed have been conscious. . . . But, by entering into connection with the unconscious tendencies during the night, they have become assimilated to the latter, degraded as it were to the condition of unconscious thoughts.
>
> (Freud, 1912, p. 265)

With regard to the metapsychology of 1915, the preconscious is not mentioned in "Instincts and their vicissitudes" (1915a) nor in "Repression" (1915b). On the other hand, the preconscious is considered both in terms of quality and system in the essay on "The unconscious" (1915c). It is there, in this attempt to arrive at a conceptual understanding that Freud presents his basic hypotheses and highlights the real problems concerning the notion of the preconscious. It is through the complexity of dividing repression into *primary repression* and *secondary repression* or *repression proper* that the topographical, dynamic and economic status of what Freud denotes by the abbreviation *Pcs.* is clarified. A system intended to promote defence, the *Pcs* uses, on the one hand, secondary repression and the withdrawal of preconscious cathexis against ideas which were once conscious, and, on the other hand, the anti-cathexis, "the sole mechanism of primal repression" (Freud, ibid., p. 181), against the unconscious ideas that have never been cathected by it before.

From this apparently somewhat tautological argument – we cannot see how or why the system *Pcs.* could and should anti-cathect an idea that it has never cathected before – we find the counterpart when Freud (ibid., pp. 178–179) speaks of the system *Cs.*: noting that repression can succeed in inhibiting an instinctual impulse from being *turned into* a manifestation of affect, he begins by deducing that "the system *Cs.* normally controls affectivity as well as access to motility" (ibid., p. 179).

However, Freud gradually went on to use more and more frequently this notation which he deliberately expressed in the form of the equation "system *Cs.*(*Pcs.*)". So, although the concept of psychic space had never been used or even clearly referred to by him since the "Project" (Freud, 1950 [1895]), I thought I could discern here, in this text of 1915 *the coexistence, in Freud's thought, of an intuition and the resistance which is attached to it*: intuition of a three-dimensional psychic space, framed by a double barrier of repression – primary repression between *Ucs.* and *Pcs.*, secondary repression between *Pcs.* and *Cs.* – and recurrent resistance, which drives him to repeat his descriptions in binary systems: *Ucs./Pcs.*, primary processes/secondary processes, free energy/bound energy, fantasy/reality. However, in the course of the text, the system *Pcs.* tends, at certain times, towards a relative degree of autonomy compared to the system *Cs.*, as evidenced by the following passages: "The processes of the system *Pcs.* display – no matter whether they are already conscious or *only capable of becoming conscious* – an inhibition of the tendency of cathected ideas towards discharge" (1915c, p. 188, my emphasis). And, further on: "[I]t devolves upon the system *Pcs.* to make communication possible between the different ideational contents, so that they can influence one other, to give them an order in time, *and to set up a censorship or several censorships*" (ibid, my emphasis). And again: "In this connection, also, we shall find means for putting an end to our oscillations in regard to the naming of the higher system which we have hitherto spoken of indifferently, sometimes as the *Pcs*, and sometimes as the *Cs*" (ibid., p. 189).

Unfortunately, when Freud speaks of the need for further research, he eradicates the third dimension from the field of the psyche and places his hopes in animal psychobiology, which allows him to fall back into a binary system with regard to psychic processes: "We must also be prepared to find possible pathological conditions under which the *two* systems [*Ucs.* and *Pcs./Cs.*] alter, or even exchange, both their content and their characteristics" (ibid., my emphasis).

So, until the end of this essay, we see Freud continuing to oscillate between two and three. In "A metapsychological supplement to the theory of dreams" (Freud, 1917b [1915], the problem of the *Pcs.* is enriched with a new element: the ego, whose status is as vague here as was that of the *Pcs.* in "Note on the unconscious in psychoanalysis" (Freud, 1912). The ego is defined here as it was in "Instincts and their vicissitudes" (1915a), that is, in terms of the ego-instincts and the first version of narcissism. The relations between the concept of the *Pcs.* and the concept of the ego in the two Freudian topographies would require a vast and detailed study, which I will not enter into here. I will limit myself to emphasizing the similarity of their respective statuses, with regard to the importance of "the penumbra of already-existing associations" (Bion, 1992, p. 73) which surrounds these two concepts in the whole of Freud's work and, perhaps, in all psychoanalytic thought. One of the two comes out of the dark – take, for instance, the *Pcs.*, erected after a fashion as a system in the first topography – while the other disappears in an artistic blur. For example, when, in *The Interpretation of Dreams*, Freud (1900) studies the effects of regression in the sleeping state, he even goes so far as to consider that the domination of the ego empties all other systems of their cathexes; but, at the same time, he describes the effects of the same regression on the *Pcs.*, *as a lowering of the censorship between Pcs. and Ucs. and an invasion of the Pcs. by the Ucs.*, leading the *Pcs.* to defend itself by means of dreams. Contrary to what would characterize the ego in the second topography – just at the moment when the *Pcs.* falls back into the adjectival penumbra – the notion of psychic work is here attached to the *Pcs.*, while the ego's narcissism aspires to absolute emptiness. However, having observed that a "dream is, therefore, also a *projection*, an externalization of an internal process", Freud (1917a [1915], p. 223) expresses his perplexity as to the reasons why projection is so important in narcissistic affections.

Freud's theorization on the differences and the similarities existing between dream and hallucination leads to a differentiation between the systems *Pcs.* and *Cs.* The hallmark of the latter is henceforth "perception" (*Pcpt.*). We realize then that this whole theorization implicitly makes the *Pcs.* system *the locus par excellence of psychic work*, concerning the exchanges between inside and outside, the subject and the world, fantasies and reality, the primary processes and the secondary processes, thing-presentations and word-presentations.

Now the fact that all of these functions of the *Pcs.* were attributed to the ego in the second topography, and that the emphasis was placed henceforth on the relations between this ego and its objects, seems to me to have played a part in diverting analytical reflection from the *preconscious status of psychic work*. The consequence of this could well be the quasi-absence, in Freud's work as a whole, of a concept of psychic space proper; such a concept cannot be logically deduced from the status of *agency* attributed to the ego in the second topography, while it was implicitly congruent with the concept of the system *Pcs.* in the first topography.

It was the problems posed by the narcissistic economy and the compulsion to repeat that made Freud switch from the first to the second topography, based entirely on the hypothesis of the death drive. And while the role of the object in the psychic economy would henceforth be recognized and studied in a masterly manner by Freud, and then by Klein and her successors, the so-called "structural" theory was to constitute a strong defence against a re-examination of the vicissitudes of the drives, a re-examination that ought to have included the death drive – that is to say the unthinkable – and the status of the objects, to which a less *realistic* situation, in the pictorial sense of the term, needed to be given than was the case in the first topography.

It must be recognized, in fact, that the role of the object is minimal in the first topography: in "Instinct and their vicissitudes", it is only considered insofar as it coincides with the aim of the drive; and is cathected and decathected at will; it is "what is most variable about an instinct and is not originally connected with it, but becomes assigned to it only in consequence of being fitted to make satisfaction possible" (Freud, 1915a p. 122).

The only obstacle to this industrial exploitation of the human object is *fixation* which, unfortunately, generally occurs "at early stages" and is solely a matter of pathology. Displacements are recognized as playing an essential role for healthy psychic functioning, but not the *quality* of the cathected objects. Moreover, the drives are also devoid of *qualitative* forms, as they are "all qualitatively equivalent".

Everything is played out in the quantitative register, until Freud is forced to reintroduce the qualitative factor in another unexplained way, in the form of the dichotomy between *sexual drives* and *ego drives*.

This journey of Freud in pursuit of the vicissitudes of the drives may make one think of an obstacle course, the obstacles being constituted by the objects. To achieve the arduous goal he set himself, that is to say how to represent the *transformations* of biological elements into psychic elements, Freud strived to simplify a problem whose extreme complexity he recognized, leaving aside the question of objects, treating them as insignificant and interchangeable for the purposes of his argument, including the object/body of the subject in auto-eroticism and the object/psyche of the subject in masochism. But the reversal of the drive into its opposite and its turning round upon the subject himself, as well as the "contrasting pairs" sadism/masochism and voyeurism/exhibitionism, would inevitably lead him to speak of "identification with an extraneous ego," to recognize that the object of voyeurism is not the eye itself, and that "in sadism, the organic source . . . points unequivocally at an object other than itself, even though that object is part of the subject's own body" (ibid., p. 132).

However, the needs of the argument cannot alone account for Freud's defensiveness on this question of the object. If he persisted in treating it as an intruder, in describing it as if it were without consistency, without resistance, without its own life within the subject, without psychic qualities on which the subject can depend affectively, it may be because he was afraid – in part consciously, moreover, if we follow this thread carefully in his correspondence – that his links with his own objects of love and hate would prevent him from fully developing his genius. Bion noted that the biggest obstacle to the achievement of "becoming what you are" – Goethe's "*Werde, was du bist*" – probably consisted in a legitimate fear of falling into megalomania and of losing contact with one's good internal objects. Following Paul Federn and Ludwig Jekels, Freud even went so far as to accomplish the feat of tackling and camouflaging in one and the same sentence the problem of the difference between the sexes:

> In the *auto-erotic* drives, the part played by of the *organic* source is so decisive that . . . the form and function of the organ determine the activity or passivity of the instinctual aim.
>
> (Freud, 1915a, p. 132–133, my emphasis)

Here, the adjective "auto-erotic" functions like dark glasses intended to reduce the glare caused by the discovery of otherness. To reduce to a *Gestalt* the question of the difference of the sexes in the human being is to try to protect oneself against the upheaval of the emotional experience of this difference, with everything that this experience brings in its wake at the level of psychic processes: projections, introjections, identifications, anxieties relating to the loss of the object, both external and internal, in the problem of the constitution of a sexual identity and psychic bisexuality.

It was in elaborating the difference between the generations – around the death of his father – that Freud came to the discovery of psychoanalysis.[2] Thus, in the double mourning that each of us faces in the resolution of our own Oedipus complex – the difference between the sexes and the difference between the generations – there is probably always one path that is more difficult than the other to tackle, even for a genius. Freud discovered the problem of mourning from the point of view of the difference between the generations, while mourning for his femininity always remained a dark continent for him, in the form of the "biological bedrock = repudiation of femininity". Is it not conceivable, as a dream if not a hypothesis, that Freud was unable to redefine the concept of the preconscious in the second topography – that is to say, in closer relation with death (death drive and mourning for the object) – because of its quality of elusive mobility which was perhaps evocative for him of femininity?

If it is to Klein that psychoanalysis owes multiple discoveries in the world of object-relations and the identifications which follow from them to, it is to Bion that credit is due for allowing us today to approach this question of the preconscious more coherently.

Starting from the Kleinian concept of projective identification, Bion established that psychic life begins in a relationship of normal projective identification occurring between the newborn baby and his mother. Thus, after the experience of what he refers to, in Freud's terminology, as the "caesura of birth", the infant can, so to speak, "expel his expulsion" and his death anxieties by projecting them into the mother's mind. These beta elements (β), which Bion (1962a) describes as "unthinkable" and which are only fit for evacuation by means of motricity, will be taken over by the mother's capacity for thinking, also called alpha function (α) or alternatively capacity for reverie, an expression, for Bion, of the drive mixture ±L, ±H, and ±K (±Love, ±Hate, and ±Knowledge). And it is here that we find, almost incidentally, the role assigned by Freud to the preconscious in the exercise of motricity: indeed, it is as if this expulsion, in the infant, occurred according to an expectant preform which elicits, in the mother, the corresponding mode of functioning, but in its elaborated form, and which is of the order of the preconscious. Let us note in passing that this particular state of mind is the very one that Freud attempts to describe under the term of "free-floating attention". Those β-elements that are not totally unthinkable for an adult mind – that is to say unrepresentable at the level of thing-presentations in the first Freudian topography – will be restored to the infant in the relationship of normal projective identification that his mother has with him, while – providing it functions well – protecting him from the reprojection of his own deadly elements, as well as from the projection of her personal death anxieties.

On the other hand, while projecting into the infant these detoxified β-elements, the mother will also project a certain quantity of α-elements, stemming from her own capacity for thinking thoughts. The gradual accretion of these α-elements in the infant's mind will form a *contact barrier*, prototypical of α-function, *which occupies the topographical locus of the Freudian Pcs.* It is from this contact barrier that unconscious fantasies will be formed, but also the system *Cs.* defined by Freud (1900) as "a sense organ for the perception of psychic qualities" (p. 615). This contact barrier, the result of the reintrojection by the infant of something in the order of the *psychic space* of the mother, will gradually function as an increasingly autonomous *internal container* for the psychic activities of the child, which form *the content*.

Thus, with his conceptualization of the "capacity for reverie" and the "contact barrier", Bion established two essential parameters which help us to better describe and understand the notion of preconscious from the Freudian perspective. Indeed, he affirms:

1 The primordial role of the mind of an external object in the constitution of a new mind.
2 The primordial role of a psychic organ – the contact barrier – *occupying the topographical locus of the system Pcs.*, in the topographical, dynamic and economic constitution of the evolving psychic apparatus.

At the same time, it makes the question of whether the drive or narcissism comes first null and void, and gives external reality a role again which takes the Kleinian model out of its apparent autarky, without falling back into the vagueness left by Freud as to the differentiation between external object and internal object. However, it should be noted that the external object considered here is *specifically the mother's mind* and not her mothering or holding activities as such. Furthermore, Bion's advances have the immense advantage of making it possible to reintroduce the model of the Freudian system *Pcs.* into the developments of the second topography, thus rendering obsolete the false dilemma of having to choose between the two Freudian topographies.

Bion considers the constitution and maintenance, within psychic life, of a "containing function" as the *sine qua non* condition of mental health and psychic development. His reflection on analytical models owes much to his study of *group phenomena* on the one hand, and *psychotic personalities* on the other. He indicates that one can observe many manifestations of the container/contained relationship in the group phenomena which take place in the "internal group" of each of the protagonists of the analytical situation. This leads him to point out that the transference on to the analyst of a parasitic mode of relating will phagocyte analyst's "container" and prevent any authentically analytic functioning, thereby leaving the content of the patient without a container. In psychotic functioning, the container is non-existent, making it impossible to differentiate between self/others, inside/outside, fantasy/reality. In borderline states, the container is both thin and distended, therefore fragile, which links up with the descriptions of the "thinness of the preconscious" mentioned in the clinical accounts of this psychic organization. Finally, in the analyst, as in the mother during her normal illness, the normal container/contained constellation, which Bion characterizes as the constellation memory/container and desire/content, must partially and voluntarily be obfuscated in order to leave room for the analogous constellation in the patient and to observe it operating at the level of the analyst's mind.

What makes the analyst's profession a high-risk profession is precisely this requirement to approach voluntarily, so closely and so often, a state of functioning of "mental illness" – even if designated as normal. As we know, the main pathological defence against such a painful state is constituted by perverse mechanisms. Conversely, the capacity for reverie, the function par excellence of the system *Pcs.*, should be increased by the exercise of analysis and contribute, in any event, to our daily safety and that of our patients.

Notes

* This text is based on the article: "Ballade au Préconscient", *Revue française de psychanalyse*, 5/1985, pp. 1391–1400 (Guignard, 1985).

1 On this subject, see Pearl King and Riccardo Steiner's *The Freud-Klein Controversies*, 1941–1945 (King & Steiner, 1991).

2 In his preface to the English translation of "Mourning and Melancholia" (Freud, 1917a [1915]) for the *Standard Edition*, James Strachey indicates that Freud's first essay on melancholia dates from 1895, that is to say, shortly before the death of his father.

Chapter 7

The unknown object of the transference

Right from the beginning of his discoveries, and in all his successive depictions of the drive economy of the human being, Freud came up against the problem of the status of the object. A grain of sand in the workings of the most elaborate formulations of Freudian thought in a constant state of evolution, the object did not succeed in establishing itself in a definitive theoretical formula any more than it constituted, in human relations studied by psychoanalytic science, an identifiable and discernible entity once and for all, except by being mortified and having a statue erected to it, like the commander in Don Juan.

From the theory of seduction to that of the threat – intensified – of castration, from the stumbling-blocks of narcissism to the paradox of the compulsion to repeat, from its modest situation as *aim of the drive* to its essential situation as the *basis of identity* through the vagaries of identification, the object constituted the ferment of all the major theoretical Freudian reorganizations. In order to maintain until the end the basic hypothesis that had already underpinned the "Project" (Freud, 1950 [1895]), according to which the human being seeks above all the satisfaction of his drives by means of discharge aimed at reducing the tension of excitation, Freud was led, as we know, to formulate new postulates on several occasions. Even when these concerned the drives (ego-drives/object-drives, life drives/death drives), or the principles of psychic functioning (pleasure principle/reality principle; systems *Ucs./Pcs./Cs.* in the first topography, id/ego/superego in the second topography) none of them can, in reality, do without this elusive element that is the object.

The shift of orientation brought about by Kleinian contributions in psychoanalytic research and clinical work led psychoanalysts to abandon the conception of the primacy of an external object indistinguishable from its support in the form of a real person in favour of that of a multiplicity of internal objects with a variety of qualities. This change of orientation made it possible to explore and describe the very many unconscious forms of object-relations, often unexpected, whose frontiers with psychotic pathology sometimes seemed slight or even non-existent. Beyond the Kleinian group, this change of orientation influenced psychoanalytic thinking as a whole; the primacy accorded to relations with internal objects gave rise in turn to a legitimate sense of perplexity concerning the role played by external reality in the constitution of the human mind.

What I am interested in here, therefore, is a perspective that takes into account the vagaries of the relationship with an object that is present as well as with an object that is absent, in external reality and psychic reality alike, which will lead me to raise the problem of the relationship to the *unknown aspects of the transference object*.

This perspective requires us, in particular, to bear in mind the following points:

1. The differentiation between the role of animate and inanimate objects or objects-things.
2. The nature of the processes of displacement permitting an inanimate object-thing to represent an animate object symbolically, following a gamut ranging from the *pictogram* to the real symbol, including the *symbolic equation* and the fetish.
3. The nature of the element which, in external reality, can link up with the primary instinctual drive expressions in order to give the infant an experience that is really of a psychic order.

Drives and affects, boundary concepts, limits of concepts

Following the introduction of the second Freudian topography, many authors would use interchangeably the concepts of "love" and "hate" as equivalents for those of the "life drive" and the "death drive", driven perhaps by the polyvalence of the concept of "libido" in the first topography. And yet, this is what Freud wrote under the aegis of the second topography:

> In psychoanalysis, no less than in other sciences, the theory of the instincts is an obscure subject. An empirical analysis leads to the formulation of two groups of instincts: the so-called 'ego-instincts', which are directed towards self-preservation, and the 'object-instincts', which are concerned with relations to an external object. . . . Theoretical speculation leads to the suspicion that there are two fundamental instincts which lie concealed behind the manifest ego-instincts and object-instincts: namely *(a)* Eros, the instinct which strives for ever closer union, and *(b)* the instinct of destruction, which leads towards the dissolution of what is living.
>
> (Freud, 1926a, p. 265)

In this article which purports to be a summary of the psychoanalytic science of the period, love and hate are not discussed explicitly. Freud only speaks of the *psychic delegation of the drives as images or ideas with an affective charge*.

Now the history of science and ideas teaches us that just as it is always in the swamp of boundary concepts that the researcher gets lost most, so it is also in these zones that he has the best chance of discovering something new. Just to give a few examples, let me cite André Green's (1973) studies on affect, whose anchor points are located in the boundary concept of the drive and in the gaps in the Freudian theory of affects; Winnicott's (1958) concept of the "good enough mother"; and finally Braunschweig and Fain's (1975) the concept of the "censorship of the woman-as-lover", with which they attempt to describe the psychic qualities of the primary object that are necessary for an initial mental organization in the infant.

My research, which is both more limited and has a slightly different orientation, also takes as its point of departure the boundary concept of the drive, and particularly the impasse in which Freud's (1915a, 1926b) recurrent position seems to leave us. In his theoretical writings, he *seems to maintain* a radical dichotomy between the drives of self-preservation and the sexual drives in the first topography, and also between the ego-drives and the object-drives in the second. This reduplication of a binary system in the space of more than ten years contains within it the sterility of the repetition-compulsion which seals every formally completed system.

On the other hand, and in parallel with this line of reasoning, Freud offers more open systems. The one he presents in "The economic problem of masochism" (Freud, 1924) seems to me to contain a richness that is commensurate with its conceptual imperfections. In it we can discern a picture of the drive system that I would call a *generational model of the drives* with, as the first generation, the life drive and the death drive; a second generation, constituted by the *pleasure/unpleasure principle*, arises from their interaction. The latter will have to unite with the "external world" in order to give rise to the *third generation*, just as fragile and under threat, namely, the *reality principle*. Thus, in the second topography, Freud reintroduces all the richness contained in "Formulations on the two principles of mental functioning" (1911), an article that itself was underpinned by the theoretical part of *The Interpretation of Dreams* (1900), in particular concerning the dream work.

Is libidinal sympathetic excitation a drive?

It is worth noting that it was at the level of this second generation of the drives that Freud would extend to suffering and unpleasure the hypothesis that he had put forward in the *Three Essays on the Theory of Sexuality*

(Freud, 1905) by postulating the appearance of a so-called "constitutional" factor which he called "libidinal sympathetic excitation". He subsequently described it as "an infantile physiological mechanism which ceases to operate later on . . . and would provide the physiological foundation on which the psychical structure of erotogenic masochism would afterwards be erected" (Freud, 1924, p. 163). Now in this reformulation of the concept of "libidinal sympathetic excitation", a concept that was a source of inspiration for the rich and familiar ideas developed by Denise Braunschweig and Michel Fain (1971) and Catherine Parat (1987), two points intrigue me: the use of the term "physiologica" l to describe such a process, and the postulate of its disappearance – one of the postulates permitting the other, logically speaking. Faced with this aporia, I will propose the following three working hypotheses:

1 Does this mechanism not also belong to the category of boundary concepts, and is it not a drive?
2 Is its so-called disappearance not due to an optical illusion, an illusion without which no researcher, even Freud, can do without when he focuses on a precise objective, in this case on the evolution of this mechanism in masochism?
3 In order to test these two first hypotheses, it is worth asking ourselves which drive it might be. This is an opportunity to wonder how Bion was able, in complete serenity, to go beyond classical Freudian duality and base his brilliant psychoanalytic theory of thinking on the drive tripod, L, H, and K, (Love, Hate, and Knowledge), drives, it must be understood, that include the entropy of each of them: ± L, ± H, ± K.

Those who have studied his work know how much importance Bion gave to the ideas developed by Freud (1911, 1900) in "Formulations on the two principles of mental functioning" and in *The Interpretation of Dreams* as well as to the discoveries of Klein between 1921 and 1945

Klein (1975) on the role, importance and aim of the epistemophilic impulses in the development of psychic life. It was precisely by reintroducing Klein's discoveries as a whole concerning the world of object relations into the package denoted by Freud (1911) as the "state of the external world" that Bion would:

1 Introduce the ego-drive constituted by the drive for knowledge (K) at the same functional level as the drives of love and hate.
2 Establish the specificity of the object, which, in this "external world", is alone capable of uniting with the pleasure/unpleasure principle of another human being in order to give birth to the reality principle in the latter. It is only a matter, of course, of a psychical quality, which he

calls the "mother's capacity for reverie", and which is the prototype of the capacity for thinking thoughts by means of a normal process of projective identification.

The reality-principle

Among the many openings this this metapsychological reorganization permits, I will mention two in connection with the subject I am dealing with:

1 The suppression of the dichotomy between ego-drives/object-drives, the three drives L, H and K being considered as being part of what I have called the *second generation of the drives*, that of the *pleasure/unpleasure principle*, which is probably specific to the human species and thus constitutes a triad of boundary concepts "drives-affects".
2 The possibility of using this triad to take a new approach to the question of the reality-principle, as Laplanche and Pontalis have written:

> It has often been asked why the child should ever have to seek a real object if it can attain satisfaction on demand, as it were, by means of hallucination. We may resolve this difficult problem by looking upon the sexual instinct as emerging from the instinct of self-preservation, to which it stands in a double relationship of both anaclisis and separation.
>
> (Laplanche & Pontalis, 1967, p. 381)

Now the drive for knowledge is unquestionably a drive of self-preservation par excellence, if indeed it is accepted that it is necessary, for one's own safety, to be aware of reality, both internal and external, in order to be able to consider whether each of these suits us or not and, if not, whether any possibilities exist to transform either or both of them, and in what way. As for the difficult question as to whether knowledge precedes the libidinal or destructive cathexis, it is one that takes us back to the imaginary dialogue between Freud and Leonardo da Vinci, which I will refer to in the next chapter.

The mother's capacity for reverie

Before offering a justification for my hypothesis concerning the parallel between Freud's idea of libidinal sympathetic excitation and Bion's K impulse and, above all, trying to understand how the latter can have such different vicissitudes as the activity of thinking, on the one hand, and masochism on the other, it is necessary to recall briefly the main outlines of Bion's theory of thinking.

For this author, thinking has its source in emotional experience, the fruit of the encounter between the infant's L, H and K impulses and the mother's capacity for reverie. This capacity for reverie depends on the mother's unconscious psychic structure, in its Oedipal and identificatory dimensions, and it is expressed in the form of dream thoughts as described by Freud. In fact, it is at the level of unconscious dream activity that *the mysterious transformation of drive activity into symbolic activity* takes place, a transformation whose causes can be suspected and effects described, but whose nature remains as unknown to us as the transformation of inert matter into living matter. Whether we approach the problem, as Freud did, from the angle of the interaction of the drives or the interaction of the pleasure/unpleasure principle and the reality principle; or whether we describe, as he did, the respective modes of functioning of thing-presentations and word-presentations; or whether we lay emphasis, with Klein, on the primordial importance of elaborating object-loss, the depressive position or the early Oedipal configuration in the advent of the capacity to symbolize; or whether, finally, we succeed, as Bion himself did, in establishing a hierarchical classification of the various modes and levels of thought, *the mystery of the advent of meaning* ultimately remains even more obscure than that of the advent of love and hate.

The most original contribution of this psychoanalytic theory of thinking certainly lies in the manner in which Bion describes the interaction of the emotional experience of thinking with other affective experiences. It enabled him to give the concept of "part-object" its full scope by extending it to *psychic functions*, the first of these objects of introjection being, precisely, the "mother's capacity for reverie". He considers that the target attacked by the subject when he seeks to destroy his own capacities for thinking and experiencing emotions is not this or that object, part or whole, internal or external in relation to the subject, but rather the *link established between objects*. It is the authentic experience of this link that permits the development of the psychical apparatus, and its somatopsychic prototype is the link between the infant's mouth and the mother's breast. Bion strictly limits the concept of "consciousness" to the definition Freud gives of it as "a sense-organ for the perception of psychic qualities" (1900, p. 615) and includes in the description of the Oedipus conflict the action of *hubris* or arrogance. Using *omnipotence* in its form of *omniscience, hubris* asserts in a dictatorial manner that one thing is morally right and the other wrong, thereby diverting the K impulse from its aim so that it henceforth risks functioning in reverse, +K becoming – K, according to one of the effects of the "negative", whose study has been developed in depth by Green (1993). Bion reverses the rationalist idea that thoughts are engendered by the activity of thinking and returns to the neo-Platonic idea that it is existing thoughts that require an apparatus for thinking them. From this point of view, and starting from the proposition that, in order to develop itself, the psychical apparatus needs *truth* just as the body needs *food*, he describes the various qualities of the process of projective identification, including in them, in distinction to the normal projective identification that constitutes the capacity for thinking thoughts, an "excessive" form of projective identification that is characteristic of the hatred of emotions and therefore, of life itself.

Truth and reality

Bion's concept of "truth" is worth dwelling on insofar as, behind its philosophical and religious appearances, it is very directly related to that of reality, a term just as uncertain but freely used in all psychoanalytic writings. And yet, who could seriously claim to be able to give a satisfying and exhaustive definition of reality in psychoanalysis, be it external reality, psychical reality, the experience of reality or the reality principle, etc., except by operating, as Jacques Lacan (1966) did, a radical cut relegating the "real" (*réel*) outside the orders of the "symbolic" and the "imaginary", thereby *turning* this reality into a real waste-product of meaning – horror? This approach may seem congruent from the logical point of view, but at the same time it gives an unreal quality to all psychic life concerning a link to the object.

Following Bion obliges us to take an equally demanding position, but in an apparently opposite direction, since horror can stem from the very discovery of meaning. Furthermore, this discovery requires an activity of thinking that is based on all the psychic qualities contained in Lacan's "symbolic" and "imaginary" orders. However, for Bion, the truth of reality does not need to be thought in order to exist.[1] It is the thinker who feel the need to find something *true* that he can gradually develop as a *thought* in his mind. Various types of relations can exist between the thought (object "O") and the thinker:

1 They may coexist in *commensalism*, that is to say without entering into relationship with one another. In other words, and if we identify with the thinker, truth, although it exists, has not been discovered.
2 Alternatively, they are in a creative relationship, in a state of *symbiosis* that modifies each of them: true thought proliferates and the thinker evolves.
3 Finally, a *parasitic relationship* is established between them, giving rise to a formulation that the thinker knows is false; he nonetheless maintains it defensively against a truth he fears because it might annihilate either the thinker/container or the true thought/content.

However, not only does Bion take it for granted that the "absolute truth" (O) can never be contained, but further that all truth requires a certain degree of falsification to be understood by the psychical apparatus. This is why he liked to point out that there is no greater liar than someone who claims he never lies.

Thus, the approach to truth by means of thinking always creates anxiety because it constitutes by definition a critical situation, which Bion calls "catastrophic change". He even regards this anxiety as the prototype of all anxiety, comparing it with the "signal anxiety" described by Freud; in so doing, he gives a more specifically psychic meaning to what Klein referred to as "death anxiety". It is this form of anxiety that underlies the mental suffering that leads the infant to defend himself against the object-loss linked to the depressive position with the radical means that characterize the paranoid-schizoid position. At its peak, the latter arouses the "nameless dread" described by Bion (1967) and the "terror of dead objects" evoked by Meltzer (1973).

Object and reality

This detour via Bion's theory allows me now to put forward a third working hypothesis, which consists in approaching the problem of reality from the angle adopted by Bion when he speaks of truth: it is plausible, I think, to consider that the relations of the psychical apparatus with external and internal reality are marked by *commensalism, symbiosis* or *parasitism* according to infinitely varying modalities. These relations are bound up with the conflict that brings love and hate into play in the interaction between the pleasure/unpleasure principle and the *drive for knowledge* (K) in the course of the emotional experiences that will generate the *reality principle.*

The forms of these relations will vary depending on the nature of the dominant psychic organization of each individual and on the degree of maturity of his psychic development. Drawing on classical nosographical structures to sketch out a brief illustration of this, it could be said that:

1 The psychotic suffers from burning hatred of the truth-of-reality, both external and psychic, against which he will build an anti-world by means of delusion and hallucinosis.
2 The pervert will use fragments of the truth-of-reality to fabricate his artificial world and will give a false formulation of it on the parasitic model of the statement, "I know, but I don't want to know", described by Freud concerning the splitting of the ego.
3 The neurotic will attempt to maintain at any price the basic assumptions of the group mentality, preferring to keep his symptoms with the

> help of repetition-compulsion rather than constantly confronting the risks of "catastrophic anxiety" linked to the activity of thinking, risks that threaten his illusory sense of coherence.

For it is necessary, in fact, to possess a considerable capacity for tolerating uncertainty and the unknown – the "negative capability" described by the poet Keats (Forman, 1952) that Bion (1970) admired so much in Shakespeare, in order to maintain in oneself, sufficiently strongly and for a sufficient length of time, the attentive availability "without memory or desire" which – perhaps one days, who knows? – will attract towards oneself a bit more truth, but at the same time turn upside down the idea that one previously had of reality.

Need I add that this "negative capability" is required both in the mother's capacity for reverie with the infant and in the psychoanalyst's free-floating attention with his patient?

Thus, driven by his impulse for knowledge and introduced to the psychic world of his projective and introjective relationship with the mother's capacity to think, the infant will progress along a ridge, at grips with love and hate *for* his objects and *of* his objects, known and unknown, absent and present.

In order to try to describe what we need to listen to in the transference, based on our countertransference, I think that it is necessary to add two approaches to the preceding discussion. The first concerns *the desire to know the present object* and the second *the relations between the impulse for knowledge (± K) and sadomasochism.*

The unknown aspects of the present object

Coinciding in this respect with Freud's assertion that "the object is known in hate" (1915a), Klein's contributions linked the appearance and functioning of epistemophilic urges to the development of sadistic impulses in the paranoid-schizoid position and, more precisely, on the threshold of the depressive position, to weaning and the onset of teething. In an earlier study, (Begoin-Guignard, 1981) I tried to dissociate these two instinctual drive expressions and suggested the importance of the quality of parental attention in the relative predominance of sadistic impulses or epistemophilic impulses in the infant.

Meltzer (Meltzer & Williams,1988) forged strong metapsychological hypotheses in connection with this question and *considered* that the aesthetic impact on the newborn infant of his first encounter with the visual world outside the uterus has been considerably underestimated. He thinks that this impact produces suffering because the newborn finds it impossible to establish any degree of correspondence between the beauty of the external aspect of the object and the nature of its hidden qualities, on the inside. He writes:

> Even at the moments of most satisfactory communication, nipple in mouth, she gives an ambiguous message, for although she takes the gnawing away from inside she gives a bursting thing which he must expel himself Truly she giveth and she taketh away, both of good and bad things. He cannot tell whether she is Beatrice or his Belle Dame de Merci. This is the aesthetic conflict which can be most precisely stated in terms of the aesthetic impact of the outside of the 'beautiful' mother, available to the senses, and the enigmatic inside which must be construed by creative imagination. Everything in art and literature, every analysis, testifies to its perseverance through life.
>
> (Meltzer & Williams, 1988, p. 22)

On the basis of this relationship to the present object, Meltzer describes *two sorts of attention*, one of which is more *active* or even intrusive, taking interest in the qualities of *the inside of the object*, and the other more *passive*, involving a movement of abandonment to the unknown, to the suffering of uncertainty, but also to the joy of the experience of an *enveloping relationship with the outside of the aesthetic object*. It is the *double identificatory relationship with the outside and the inside of the present object* that constitutes what he calls "aesthetic conflict", a conflict that he sees as the *very essence of depressive position*.

Sadomasochism as a defence against knowing the object

My second approach concerns the implications of this separation of the epistemophilic impulses from the sadistic impulses for the organization of sadism and masochism as classically described. We could thus consider that *sadism*, oral then anal, which, as we know, constitutes one of the most usual defences of love and hate against the object, is not directed so much against the absence of an object that was previously felt to be satisfying, but rather against the upheaval due to the discovery that there is *too great a discrepancy between the external and internal aspects of the object*.

Such was the case with a female patient whose abundant and complicated material had required great attention and intense analytic activity from me during the whole session and who, the following day, told me how happy she felt about her experience in the session the day before, but at the same time was terribly disappointed that I had used the word "work" to refer to what had happened between us.

The double turning around of the drive – into its contrary and against the subject's own self – which, classically, defines masochism, may equally be considered as the other side of a *parasitic relationship with the truth/reality of the object*. The double identificatory relationship with the outside and inside of the object will assume an overly intrusive quality, projective identification will become pathological, the drive impulse K will be denied or foreclosed, and the economic principle of masochism will operate efficiently, since masochism remains the most impenetrable defence against taking cognizance of the beauty of the otherness of the object.

Drawing on the various arguments presented earlier, I can now put forward the following hypotheses: the more the infant's relationship with the enveloping outside of the primary object has been disturbed, the more the means of defence involving projective identification with this impaired container is likely to be intense and pathological. This will give rise to a mode of cathexis classically described as masochistic, because the support of a K cathexis to the L and H cathexes concerning this container, of feminine valency for the unconscious, is lacking. In other words, this will result in a pathological identification of the subject with a pseudo-femininity.

If, on the contrary, the discovery of the *inside of the object* has aroused anxieties that are too intense to permit the K impulse to be supported by L and H in its penetrating relationship with the object, the pathological expression will be located more in the domain of *sadism*, through pathological projective identification with the object which avoids being penetrated.

The unknown dimension of the object in the analytic relationship

As a psychoanalyst, it is obvious to me that the problem of the status of the object in the analytic relationship must be approached from the angle of situations in which my countertransference allows me to identify this object as a transference object, otherwise I would lose, if not my soul, then my identity as an analyst – and perhaps that amounts to the same thing. What I can say about the object is derived only from perception, often more affective than ideational, from something that occurs in the fragile moment of the meeting between an instinctual drive expression and the transference. And it is only my countertransference that has the power to bring to this situation the third dimension that gives it substance.

A female patient was considering ending a long analysis that had often been difficult due to persistent depressive moods and masochism that protected her against mourning her Oedipal objects. Having finally rediscovered a certain joy in living, she was concerned about her rediscovered liveliness and the simple and serene pleasure she had in doing the ordinary things of life, but also about her greater capacity to accept the inevitable share of sadness and restriction involved in recognizing the reality principle. In this state of mind, she suddenly thought again about a fantasy that had featured throughout her analysis in which she saw herself hampered in clothes which she expected me to free her from. At the same time, she felt terrified because she was convinced that I would be unable to do this without tearing off her skin in the process: "Today," she said, "I would really like to know what *you* think about it".

I asked her if she remembered what thoughts we had had about this image.

HER – You told me that, even in the sarcophagi I was talking about, there were grains that grew when one took them out of there and let them germinate. . . . But for skin?

ME – You were unable to get out of your father's skin without feeling that you were tearing off your own.

HER – But why my father? Is it because we have to begin at the end?

ME – Because, once you had unstuck yourself from him, you did not feel able to enter into maternal intimacy; today, it seems that you can.

HER – It looks as if I'm less afraid of encountering terrifying things there . . . dead, perhaps?

ME – Perhaps it has also become a place that is less forbidden for you to know . . .

HER – Today, I feel like walking around in the middle of everything you have proposed me during this analysis . . . as if I was at home!

She laughed, and then spoke about projects, feeling on the edge of something new that she was not as yet able to undertake. Would she have the desire, the strength of desire?

She remarked, smiling: "I need a rattle!" Then she associated to a story of phimosis in which the man who had been operated on feared that his foreskin might disappear along with the bandage when it was removed!

This short passage from an ordinary session illustrates, I think, one of the major aspects of the Oedipal configuration in the girl, in a movement in which the latter ceases to identify projectively with a dead father and can attribute a functional role to penis envy in the organization of her inverted Oedipus complex. We can see the end of the analysis emerging, with a real reintrojection of living and differentiated parental imagos or, in other words, the subjectivation of the transference objects.

A male patient discovered, after long years of analysis, that psychic space is more suited to dealing with problems of development and thought than is the body and somatization, of which he had hitherto been an undisputed champion. At the same time, he began to get a glimpse, not without a sense of dread, of the possibility of freeing himself from a false-self that both concealed and protected a rich personality, but one that was still on the frontiers of early childhood psychically speaking. During a session when he showed he was capable, perhaps for the first time, of tolerating a considerable regressive movement while continuing to verbalize what he was experiencing, he told me, in dream-like state:

HIM – I feel inhabited by a parasitic object; it could be X, a child who died before I was born and whom my mother grieved over unduly, even though it was only the son of her best friend. I experience this X like a double; which of us is the aborted child? Then it becomes a gang, a form of gangrene; "they" are a group, a hubbub . . . and then there's a total absence of thought; emptiness.

ME – As if they had taken your thoughts with them when leaving you?

HIM – (*very excited, barely letting me finish my sentence*) Around my baby bottle? It's a real scalp dance! (He suffered from severe eating disorders during the first weeks of his existence).

He suddenly fell asleep for a few moments. When he woke up, I said to him:

ME – From hyperexcitation to anaesthesia, there was no one to accompany you.

HIM – Yes, no desire. I've always had the same attitude towards desire: The initial experience is one of trembling, a sort of bedazzlement; either it takes shape a long time after or not at all, there's nothing between the two. . .

Suddenly terrified, he continued:

HIM – It happened suddenly: one night, when I was a child, I had the impression I was being penetrated, infiltrated, fucked by something that had proliferated, installed itself, eaten me and lived at my expense . . . was it my father? Was it homosexuality? It seems very clear to me and yet this is the first time I have formulated it like that. . . . I remember, we were living in X, so I was three or four years old: it was as if I had been kidnapped and returned afterwards, but it was no longer me. . . . If I had not been returned at all, it would've been easier, but instead a lethal double was returned that was only able to develop itself at my expense . . .

It would be quite wrong to take this moment of awareness for a delusional movement. At the very most, one could speak here of a progressive hallucinatory movement thanks to which this patient managed to give shape to, and to imagine, some of his internal objects, in particular, the internal object of his melancholic maternal object (X, the dead child), and his internal paternal object with whom he had hitherto been merged to the point of suffering physically from the organic destruction of his dead father. Here, the transference object is not to be identified among these proliferating and parasitic objects. Indeed, at no moment did the patient feel persecuted by my presence. He stayed at a cautious distance from me, observing with astonishment my desire to listen to him with as much tact and attention as possible. There was a genuine analytic intimacy between us, but it resided exclusively in the care I took to recognize the validity of the meaning that he was looking for in extremely old and precise memories, but ones that were still denied by a family circle that had only attributed a physical existence and not a psychical existence to him. However, this meaning could not have come to light had I not considered myself from the beginning of the analysis as a reliable receptacle for psychic suffering that he himself was unaware of, identified as he was with the numbing and multiple splitting of his internal parental objects. For him, it was not a matter of reconstructing historicity archaeologically, but rather of making it emerge through a primary relationship of reverie. It was as if since the very beginnings of his existence he had given up any hope of making himself understood, and for a very long time he pretended that I was just as mad as him because I was struggling to understand what had seemed insignificant for many others. The fragment that I have reported here marked a decisive turning-point in the analysis, after which he accepted me as a memory of this episode, which he began by forgetting totally, being able henceforth to rely on the fact that I was going to remember it. Instead of his hypermnesia of the distant past and his total forgetting of the session of the day before, we witnessed the simultaneous organization in him of normal repression and immediate memory. A genuine dialogue was established, with me, but above all with himself. It seems to me that the transference object here is the object/witness of a new life, an object whose metaphor might be a parental couple leaning over a cradle, amazed by this life that is different from their own and whose evolution they will have the privilege of following with respect and love for its otherness.

Reverie

We are trapped by words. And particularly those we use with the aim of describing a living phenomenon that unfolds and deploys itself in a psychic space/time. They could very well be reified in the very movement in which we try to make abstract concepts of them. It is unlikely that I will be able to avoid this trap totally as I try to circumscribe the *unknown object of the transference.*

In the clinical fragments presented earlier, I tried to identify this unknown object in its "unbearable lightness" (Kundera, 1984), the ephemeral instant in which it becomes knowable thanks to the triple drive link L, H, and K rediscovered by the analyst in the conflictual chaos of the analysand's internal objects. Depending on the cases and the moments, the destiny of the transference object will be to constitute a transitional object in place of a fetishistic object: "I need a rattle", joked the *female patient;* or, "to envelop the ego", as we may suppose for the *male patient* in the preceding account of the session. Whether it is called an "anaclitic object (Freud), a "psychic envelope" (Anzieu), a "stimulus barrier" (Fain and Braunschweig), or a "containing object" (Bion), in every case, the transitory function of the transference object, each time it reveals itself, will be in the nature of transformation through repetition, as the following lines from Verlaine suggest:

> Often I have this strange and penetrating dream of a
> Woman unknown, whom I love and who loves me;
> She is different every time, never quite the same,
> Never wholly changed; she loves and understands me.
>
> Paul Verlaine, 1866, *Poèmes saturniens* [Saturnine Poems, VI (Verlazza, 2019]

The internal objects that make our analysand's suffer are dead, faecalized, inert and useless objects and, as such, invasive and persecuting. The mourning of such objects, immobilized in their eternity, is impossible because only living objects can be used to produce introjections that are really identificatory in the post-Oedipal sense in which Freud used this term. To return to his argument, the ego of our patients must be able, in the transference relationship, to find these drive links L, H and K which will reanimate their dead objects and permit the *ego* finally to leave them to their past and to follow its own destiny, present and future.

As a woman analyst, my identity gives its shape to my discourse: concerning the transference objects identified in my clinical examples, I did not explicitly comment on the aspect of the castration complex or that of homosexuality, even though they are evident; instead I chose formulations that were more spontaneously organized around concepts expressing the links that may exist between the masculine and the feminine. In the cathexis of ordinary bisexuality, the analyst at work seems to me to be particularly challenged at the level of his feminine position, his capacity to receive and to contain emotions linked to the memory traces of another human being in order to restore them to him in more living dimensions. I will recall here my suggestion[2] that masochism and femininity should be considered as standing together in a Moebius strip relationship, and I would like to mention in this connection the anecdote used by physicists when trying to help the uninitiated understand what the quantum object is:

> An optimistic fisherman cast his line into a pond that was so muddy that no one could tell what was in it. He was rewarded for his curiosity because he soon felt a fish biting on his hook. He thus inferred, logically, that the fish was swimming around in the pond in search of food. But unlike the physicist [and, I would add, the psychoanalyst], it

> would never have had the idea that before biting on the hook, the fish was only a sort of fish potentiality occupying the whole pond.
> (Ortoli & Pharabod, 1984, p. 67, translated for this edition)

A new meaning for the primal scene, arising from the infantile Oedipal organization, will emerge from the integration of psychic bisexuality when adult biological capacities come into play. The primal scene will then become the organizing fantasy of adult sexuality, in a psychic space structured both by the transgenerational vector of the parental function and by the generational vector of the loving relationship. The first of these vectors will retain its restrictive character throughout life – a telescoping of the generations excepted. The second will retain its random character, since it concerns the relationship between couples.

The delimitation of the field in which the transference objects can reveal themselves will arise from the coming together of these two vectors. Only the transfero-counter-transferential analytic relationship will permit the transformation of the potentiality of transference objects which, like the physicist's fish potentiality occupies the whole muddy pond of the unconscious until the fisherman/analyst enables it to take shape. As for this object/fish, I cannot impress strongly enough on fisherman that our attention must be both dreamy and sustained, for no one knows where and when the fish will take shape, and there are many species.

Notes

1 This is reminiscent of Galileo's remark when, obliged to repudiate his astronomical theories concerning the earth's orbital revolution and to burn his work, he grumbled, it is said: *"Eppur, si muove!" – And yet, it turns!*

2 See the chapter "Le sourire du chat" (1986) in my book *Épître à l'objet* (Guignard, 1997a).

Chapter 8

Leonard and Sigmund

Love, hate and knowledge

In the extraordinary psychoanalytic novel "Leonardo da Vinci and a memory of his childhood", Freud (1910) tackles the mysteries of the processes of sublimation in relation to genius. His conclusions have already given rise to a very abundant literature (Klein, 1923; Chasseguet-Smirgel, 1967; Barande, 1977; Green, 1993), but it is not my purpose to take stock of it or comment on it here. For my part, I wish to examine a problematic though well-defined aspect of the question, resulting from the description made by Freud of the *three vicissitudes of drive energy in sublimation.*

Throughout this text, we see Freud grappling with the statement that he was already well-familiar with, situating the origin of curiosity in children at around the age of 3, at the time of "infantile sexual researches" and in relation to the discovery that another child could be born after him. Having recalled that the wave of repression will soon enough overcome the flood of questions asked by the child of this age instead of the only one he will never ask – where do children come from? – Freud explores further the evolution of infantile curiosity. He distinguishes, first of all, two neurotic vicissitudes:

1 The first, in which infantile sexual researches give way entirely to repression, suggests an aetiology for mild intellectual impairment that has since been verified (Guignard, 1972).
2 The second is where "intellectual development is strong enough to resist the sexual repression which has hold of it" but where "the interminable character of the child's researches is also repeated" and leads to "compulsive brooding", evokes the compromise between curiosity or the urge to know and obsessive mechanisms.

And it was Leonardo, clearly representing the mystery that his own genius posed for Freud, who would lead Sigmund to postulate a third vicissitude for the evolution of the libido and to write the most disconcerting lines on the subject of sublimation:

> The third type, which is the rarest and most perfect, escapes both inhibition of thought and of neurotic compulsive thinking. It is true that here too sexual repression comes about, but it does not succeed in relegating a component instinct of sexual desire to the unconscious. Instead, *the libido evades the fate of repression by being sublimated from the very beginning into curiosity [Wissbegierde]* and by becoming attached to the powerful instinct for research *[Forschertrieb]* as a reinforcement. Here too, the research becomes to some extent compulsive and a substitute for sexual activity; but, owing to the complete difference in the underlying psychical processes (sublimation instead of an irruption from the unconscious) the quality of neurosis is absent; there is no attachment to the original complexes of infantile sexual research, and *the instinct can operate freely in the service of intellectual interest*. Sexual repression, which has made the instinct so strong through the addition to it of sublimated libido, is still taken into account by the instinct, in that it avoids any concern with sexual themes.
>
> (Freud, 1910, p. 105, my emphasis)

In the rest of the text, Freud only develops the line of a "part instinct of sexual pleasure/desire", the *Wissbegierde* which Ilse Barande (1977, p. 74) stresses is an ordinary term in German and translates fairly well as "yearning, or urge to know", which, she adds, "restores its sensual and imperative dimensions". On the other hand, while studding his text with words from the family of *Forschung* – research – he does not really return to this "*Forschertrieb*", this "instinct for research", whose existence immediately seems so obvious to him, although he does not assign any clearly defined status to it in his theorization of the libido.

Before attempting to address the possible reasons for such an avoidance, let us return to the pages of striking beauty in which Freud establishes an imaginary dialogue with Leonardo on the vicissitudes of love, hatred and knowledge. This dialogue aims, at the level of conscious intent, to introduce his theory as to the reasons that led Leonardo to be interested more and more in science, gradually abandoning the plastic arts under the effect of an inhibition that supposedly hampered his artistic creativity. In support of his thesis, Freud brings together testimonies concerning the daring manner, at once extraordinarily thorough and meticulous, with which Leonardo carried out his preliminary researches, and the irresolute, inhibited manner – dare I say phobic? – with which he worked on his definitive works:

> LEONARD – One has no right to love or hate anything if one has not acquired a thorough knowledge of its nature. . . . For great love

> springs from great knowledge of the beloved object, and if you know it but little you will be able to love it only a little or not at all; in truth, great love is born from great knowledge of the object loved, and if you know something just a little, you will be able to like it just a little or not at all.
>
> (Leonardo da Vinci (c. 1490–1519), *A Treatise on Painting*, I, 64, p. 54, in Freud, 1910, p. 73)

> FREUD – It is not true that human beings delay loving or hating until they have studied and become familiar with the nature the object to which these affects apply; on the contrary, they love impulsively, from emotional motives which have nothing to do with knowledge, and whose operation is at most weakened by reflection and consideration.
>
> (Freud, 1910 p. 74)

In this passionate protest by Freud, one cannot fail to be struck by the contrast between the violence of the exclamation and the bitterness of the comedown; and also, by this denial that any positive relationship exists between feelings and the desire to know. And particularly in a text that introduces a new dimension to this desire – a dimension which, it is true, remains in the state of a mere observation, even though it is part of the very object of the Freudian discoveries that are the drives. Besides, a few pages later, Freud confides further:

> Because of his insatiable and indefatigable thirst for knowledge [*Forscherdrang*], Leonardo has been called the Italian Faust. But quite apart from doubts about a possible transformation of the instinct to investigate [*Forschertrieb*] back into an enjoyment of life – a transformation which we must take as fundamental in the tragedy of Faust – the view may be hazarded that Leonardo's development approaches the Spinoza's mode of thinking. A conversion of psychical instinctual force into various forms of activity can perhaps no more be achieved without loss than a conversion of physical forces. The example of Leonardo teaches us how many other things we have to take into account in connection with these processes. The postponement of loving until full knowledge is acquired ends in a substitution [*Ersatz*] of the latter for the former. A man who has won his way to a state of knowledge cannot properly be said to love and hate; he remains beyond [*jenseits*] love and hatred. He has investigated instead of loving. And that is perhaps why Leonardo's life was so much poorer in love than that of other great men, and of other artists. The stormy passions of a nature that inspires and consumes, passions in which other men have enjoyed their richest experience, appear not to have touched him. There are some further consequences. Investigating has taken the place of acting and creating as well.
>
> (Freud, 1910, p. 75]

Such an opposition between curiosity and joy of living, between knowledge of the object and love/hate for it – insofar, moreover, as it already announces "Beyond the pleasure/unpleasure principle" and therefore, the second Freudian topography – can only be understood from a perspective in which the elaboration of the Oedipus complex stalls doubly on account of the overly painful loss of the parents of early infancy.

The whole *childhood memory* – starting with its title – could be heard, analytically speaking, as the expression of the suffering of the child Sigismund who, in order to develop, had to leave the "narcissistic elation" dear to Béla Grunberger (1971) for the valley of tears of the depressive position, as described by Klein, with the introjective necessity of working through the experience of mourning for the lost object. It can also be heard in terms of Freud's ambivalent position with regard to his own latent homosexuality, projected onto that of Leonardo. The smiling and eclectic genius of Leonardo, passing with disconcerting ease from art to science, making visible without words the invisible dimension of things, may very well have aroused a certain nostalgic jealousy in Freud, whose intangible object of research and discovery could only lead him to feel disillusioned about the habitual evolution in human beings of this fabulous vital force that is the libido. The opposition that Freud sets up between research and creation constitutes, does it not, the *negative side of the feeling of admiration* that Freud always expressed towards great artists? Of course, such a question must remain unanswered. It merely reminds us that, if they are to be bearable, the narcissistic wounds of each of us must be integrated coherently into our development. Little is known about those of Leonardo, apart from his illegitimacy which he seems to have always casually denied, taking over with authority the name of a father that was also the name of his birthplace. At most, they may be seen as the negative underside of the happy and loving words that the painter holds out to his students in his prodigious *Treatise on Painting* (da Vinci, 1651): could this joy in loving, which Leonardo sees as depending on the joy of knowing, not also be understood as an elaboration of his Oedipal conflict and as a triumph of love over hate towards a father whose reckless fatherhood he forgave once he had got to know him better? Does it not constitute, for this Master who taught so many young people, an ideal narcissistic model? So, beyond the manifest homosexual aspect, does this model not lead us straight towards a primitive scene fantasy that includes a mother who had derived lasting satisfaction from having loved the one who, according to the equation mentioned by Freud at the beginning of his text, had given her his penis in the form of this prodigious son?

The links established by Freud between the homosexual structure of Leonardo and the pathological aspects of a painting inhibition which, in spite of everything, was never total and did not prevent him from becoming one of the greatest creators and discoverers of all the times are, certainly, interesting, but seem to me to "miss the point" sketched out by the author at the beginning of his study. Is it really necessary to follow Freud's affirmations concerning the crippling antagonism that exists, in his view, between the instinctual offshoots of love and hatred on the one hand and of the urge to know on the other, in spite of the fact that Leonardo seems to demonstrate the contrary? Can we not hear here something of another order, that of a *fantasy of transgression* which plagued Freud throughout his revolutionary discoveries and that he disguised by making the thirst for knowledge an unsatisfactory substitute for the impulse to love? In support of this idea, let us recall what he was to write ten years later, in *Beyond the Pleasure Principle*:

> The difference in amount between the pleasure of satisfaction which is demanded and that which is actually achieved that proves the driving factor which will permit of no halting at any position attained, but, in the poet's words, "*ungebändigt immer vorwärts dringt*" ("Presses ever forward unsubdued", Mephistopheles, Faust, Part I Scene 4)
>
> (Freud, 1920, p. 42)

I would like to suggest that, in his eagerness to write about Leonardo, Freud repressed the idea of an *instinct for research* for reasons of guilt. He was certainly not fooled by the transferential and identificatory relationship that guided his research, passionate and meticulous too, to find meaning in the life of this other of himself who was the genius Leonardo. Writing about Leonardo, Goethe or Michelangelo was a means for Freud of approaching his own genius through fraternal intermediaries, and so to recognize it in spite of himself.

It was also a way of putting himself in a situation of comparison, and even of rivalry with them. There is a considerable contrast between Freud's insightful analysis of Leonardo's character and his clumsy construction, both on the subject of his infantile history and of his excessively famous childhood memory of it. It is as if he absolutely wanted to make Leonardo a fatherless child in early childhood, when there is no evidence that Caterina and her baby really lived outside the geographical radius of Ser Piero, whose son Leonardo always recognized himself as, despite his illegitimacy.

Not wishing to venture in turn hazardous hypotheses, I will simply point out that Sigismund, the first child of a third marriage, had many reasons to feel rivalry, both with his two elder half-brothers and with his nephew of the same age, as well as with little Julius: the latter had robbed him of the comfort of his mother's physical presence when Sigi was only seven months old – therefore, certainly, following his weaning and the return of Amalia's menstrual periods – and later died, precisely, at the age of 7 months. Faced with such an avalanche of Oedipal rivals of such diverse ages and destinies, how could he not dream a little of the lost paradise of undivided maternal love, and attribute to Leonardo – his "brother in genius" – a long intimacy with his mother, when he himself had been deprived so early from such intimacy? How could he not take revenge by asserting, without evidence and by way of deploring it, the absence of an Oedipal father in Leonardo? And, above all, how could he not subtly express his rivalry by using the fruit of his own genius – his discovery of psychic processes – to interpret in his own way and with an authority that brooked no questioning, what Leonardo had written on the role of love and hate in knowledge? However, more than to such arguments, which are perhaps debatable, the reader today will certainly be sensitive to the immense disillusionment and acute suffering of the little Sigi who was still palpitating in the interpretation by the great Sigmund of Leonardo's smiling affirmations.

From the Italian Faust to the Viennese Faust via the German Faust, there is only a small distance, which we can allow ourselves to cover: does not Freud himself mention one of Goethe's childhood memories, in a 1919 note added to *Leonardo*, recalling the equally vehement protest of the little Johann Wolfgang breaking dishes, without associating this anger with the birth of a little brother – which Freud does not fail to notice, even though he forgets "his" own Julius!

I would like to focus here on this potential space opened up by Freud's refutation of Leonardo's remarks on the convivial relations that exist between love, hate and knowledge. I will, of course, avoid another pitfall which would be to try to offer an answer to another millennial question. I will content myself with examining the *problem of the part played by sadistic impulses in the urge to know*. Indeed, Freud's painful remarks cannot fail to direct our attention implicitly to the complex entanglement of sadism in the processes of introjection and, consequently, of knowledge of the object. Klein (1932) made oral-sadistic and anal-sadistic impulses the first instinctual drive impulses expressing simultaneously, in phantasy life, the fear of losing the object and the frantic desire to retain it at all costs – even by tearing into the breast or by wildly forging a passage through the anus towards the inside of the mother's body, a place idealized in sensory memory (Mancia, 2007) as containing all the riches lost by the child at his birth. She subsequently regarded this "phase of exacerbated sadism", which she located around the end of the first six months of life, as the "threshold of the depressive position", and always maintained the idea that it was at this juncture that, almost simultaneously, the *subject-object differentiation and the recognition of the existence of the third party* – object of the object, paternal object of a first Oedipal triangulation – appear under the increased organizing influence of genital impulses. While leaving us admirable observations and irreplaceable theoretical parameters on the instinctual drive impulses and object relationships of infants, Klein (1952) did not, however, offer a distinct conceptual status for the epistemophilic impulses.

I nevertheless think that one could consider "envy", this determination to destroy beauty, goodness or, more simply, the efficacy of the object that one cannot possess, a concept of which Klein (**1957**) paints a terrible and masterful description in her last written work, as the expression of an alliance between the sadistic impulses and the *negative of the instinct for research (Forschertrieb)* of which Freud speaks – Bion's minus K.

Bion (1962a), on the other hand, unhesitatingly adopted this position sketched out by Freud in *Leonardo* and which makes *the instinct for research* – or *the urge to know* – if not a drive in its own right, at least, a first drive offshoot, on the same level as love and hate, if one insists, as I do, on preserving the frontier status of the concept of drive. From this triad, it is therefore important to examine how this drive is articulated, on the one hand, with the individual development of narcissistic and object-cathexes, and on the other with group mentality, which so often makes use of its negative aspect. We could, currently, use the subsequent discoveries of Freud (1940 [1938]) on the ego-splitting and those of Klein (1946) on the splitting of the object to attempt a re-reading of Freud's description of the character of Leonardo: if the human subject remains in this idealized vision of the happy union of love and knowledge, it can only be at the cost of *splitting* off hate, which plays such a constricting role in everything that constitutes the desire for possession in the form, precisely, of sadistic, oral and anal impulses.

A subtle trace of this can be noted, moreover, in the first part of the beautiful declaration of Leonardo, quoted by Freud (1910), which includes hatred: "One has no right to love *or hate* anything if one has not acquired a thorough knowledge of its nature" (p. 73, my italics). Until then, hatred of the object had been seen as one of the possible outcomes of the process of knowledge. But the rest of the text eliminates the problem so as to focus only on love. One could therefore argue that once indifference has been superseded by ignorance or misappraisal, either the object is loved or it is split by Leonardo who, with smiling bonhomie, rejects hated objects into the *nowhere* of an outside world which does not concern him more. At the same time, ambivalence, considered by Freud as the result of an evolution towards genitality, disappears from the picture, if I may put it that way.

Now, thus projected into the outside world by the subject who, consequently, no longer has control of them within his individual psychic organization, sadistic impulses are likely to take terrible revenge on the beauty of the union of love and knowledge, by allying itself, in the form of envy, with the tremendous destructiveness contained in the group mentality and expressed by "the primitive horde" described by Freud (1912–1913). Such is the fate of the works of genius, for we know how difficult and ineffective it has always been to protect them against iconoclasts.

To return to the field of individual psychology, we find much evidence of the harmful effects of this splitting on the libidinal economy of artists. We can therefore only recognize the merits of the Freudian ideal of ambivalence, as well as of the Kleinian requirement for integrative work on sadistic impulses in the economic equilibrium of the subject: however imperfect it is, their internal elaboration at the level of the organization of secondary repression must serve as a phase of decompression in the face of envious attacks, internal and external. That said, is Freud's bitterness about the loss of the ability to love the known object inevitable? We find ourselves here, it seems to me, at one of the frontier zones between the potentiality of individual psychic development and the historicity of the family, transgenerational and social situation in which the individual was born. In other words, while all destinies are constrictive, even for geniuses, they are not all so in the same way.

Thus we may suppose that Leonardo fully used his situation as an illegitimate child, albeit living under the paternal roof, on the one hand to make this generous and unconventional father a model with whom he could identify in the field of teaching painting – not all painters strive so generously to look for ways of transmitting their technique – and, on the other hand, to maintain his status as a wonderful child, freed both from material pressures and from the worry of making a place for himself in the society of the time. Dedicating all his energy to the deployment of his genius, he seems to have transcended, for many years and without any apparent effort, the shame and guilt linked to his status as an illegitimate child, by achieving social recognition to the extent of becoming a celebrity. One might therefore assume that splitting, the basic mechanism allowing human beings to defend against the primary state of confusion, was used by Leonardo to the best of the opportunities available to him. However, this psychological situation of splitting has its limits, especially when it is operative in an unusual personality. We can indeed observe in gifted subjects – and, all the more so in geniuses – a particularly flexible and subtle balance between good capacities of "healthy" splitting, which allow them not to lose their instinctual drive energy in useless brooding, and exceptionally strong integrative ego trends, which allow them to preserve their internal coherence. It is reasonable therefore to wonder whether the inhibition detected by his contemporaries in Leonardo and attributed by Freud to the return of repressed sexuality cannot be understood as a long-term failure of the effectiveness of the splitting mechanisms which had served so well at the start of his awesome development. Thus "caught up", as it were, by the internal negative factors which he had for so long evacuated into the outside world without any evident persecutory return, Leonardo finally felt over the course of time – more normally one might say – more threatened by his audacity in deploying under the gaze of others his highly exceptional gifts.

In presenting to the world discoveries as scandalous as those of the unconscious and infantile sexuality, and having to struggle perpetually for recognition in the Viennese milieu, without any financial support, how could Freud have had such a narcissistic vision of his own genius as Leonardo had, at least until near the end of his life? Freud also used this harsh reality of his own as best he could to work towards the integration at an Oedipal level of his sadistic impulses, while working hard for the transmission of his knowledge, on a traditional millennia-old identificatory basis that was very different from that of Leonardo. Though it was sad for him that he had to pay the price for it by believing he had lost his capacities to love the known object, we can only admire the fact that he was able, at the same time, to feel he was beyond the hatred of which he was both the witness as a child – in the episode of the father's cap, for instance – and the object as an adult, in a world gone mad under the rise of Nazism.

The aim of sadistic impulses is twofold: linked to greed and intolerance of frustration, they aim to recover at all costs the omnipotent possession of the object; linked to envy, they paralyze the development of the ego by ransacking the object that is unavailable for absolute possession.

The aim of the urge for knowledge is twofold: linked to feelings of distress and infantile helplessness, it seeks to explore the interior of the object in order to discover elements of meaning that can be given to the subject's suffering; linked to love for the object, it sensually explores its characteristics which will serve as a support for the subject's identifications.

In my opinion, the role of parental objects, first external and then internalized, is crucial for the establishment of a formal representation, even if it is not always achievable, of a possible balance between a good development of the urge for knowledge and a sufficiently unruffled approach to sadistic impulses in the infant. For this, a certain quality of non-projective attention seems essential, and it is perfectly logical that Freud perceived his loss during the subsequent pregnancy of his mother. The remarkable thing is that he retained the impression that led him to see in it the libidinal origin of the desire for knowledge, and even the intuition of this "urge to know", which he mentions, without using it on a theoretical level, in *Leonardo*. You will remember that I suggested that a repression had occurred in Freud, while he was writing under the effect of unconscious guilt, of this intuition which was nonetheless important from the point of view of libido theory. If my hypothesis is correct, the repression was due to the concomitant emergence of his sadistic impulses, which he had to work over alone, in a state of infantile distress that one can well imagine. Did he not write: "A mother's love for the infant she suckles and cares for is something far more profound than her later affection for the growing child"? (Freud, 1910, p. 117).

The oldest reason for his bitter remarks about the fate of the known object may well lie therein.

The fusion of the sadistic impulses and the urge to know gives rise to extremely diverse clinical pictures, depending on the instinctual drive aim sought afte:

When sadistic impulses predominate, the pleasure obtained is above all organ pleasure, where auto-eroticism develops without concern for the object of satisfaction, or else, a pleasure of performance where interest in competition prevails over interest in the aim to be achieved, or even a pleasure of omnipotent control over the object, used for perverse ends, whether acted out or not. In all cases, the repetition-compulsion is predominant and not very developmental, in that it aims exclusively at ensuring a reductive narcissistic satisfaction which constantly thwarted because of the means used and the importance of the destructive attacks against living objects of identification. In the best of cases, the taste for material possessions, for allegedly irrefutable evidence and for scientific models devoid of creative hypotheses all seem to me to fall into this category. Disruptions in the balance of this mode of organization give rise to depressive states that are difficult to recover from, all understanding and insight gained in the analytic treatment being immediately prey to the subject's faecalizing envy towards it. The negative therapeutic reaction constantly threatens the therapeutic alliance and, when real progress nevertheless occurs, anxiety is strongly reactivated by any change. Such change is experienced as a threat of loss of control over the object/prey as well as over aspects of the subject which have received developmental elements from it in order to introject them.

When the urge to know prevails over the sadistic impulses, the pleasure obtained is a pleasure of the psyche-soma as a whole, of the activity of imagination, so dear to Leonardo, of discovery and creativity, passionately pursued, both by him and by Freud, despite the latter's disillusioned reflections on the misadventures of the man who loved.

The *pathology of splitting* can moreover offer support for such hypotheses, on account of its overriding importance in the failures that one can observe concerning the fusion of the sadistic impulses with the epistemophilic impulses. The fine work of Janine Chasseguet-Smirgel (1967) on true and false creativity is evidence of this. From neurosis to perversion, from inhibitions of thought to mental debility, from hypochondria to psychosomatic illnesses and from schizophrenia to paranoia, the study of disorders of splitting can be conducted with reference to the effect of its pathology on the confusion existing between the urge to know and the sadistic impulses, between the desire for research and voyeurism, between real thought-processes and pseudo-intellectual padding, between creative imagination and false originality.

Chapter 9

The countertransference of the adult analyst

In the light of the transference of the child in analysis

Transference in the child

Gone are the days, it seems to me, when the existence of transference in the child was subject to doubt. Anna Freud remains the emblematic figure of the path travelled in this domain: in 1927, she denied that a child could form a real transference; in 1965, she recommended the analysis of the said transference. From whatever horizon they come, all those who have had children in analytic treatment recognize today that transference in the child exists and can legitimately be cited, recognized and interpreted.

Moreover, it is surprising retrospectively that so many analysts were able to deny for such a long time that the child has a capacity to transfer, when our entire theoretical corpus is based on the discovery of infantile sexuality and the Oedipus complex. If access to the Oedipal configuration implies the acquisition of the capacity to establish a triangulated network of relationships – thus to cathect a new, non-fusional object, one might say – it has to be recognized that this process sets in very early on in the young infant, failing which, the first psychic development, and in particular the incipient stages of language and meaning, could quite simply not take place.

A child's transference is intense, extremely polymorphous, and often concealed by phobic reactions. Its intensity, both positive and negative, will be expressed all the more through acting out in that the instinctual drive excitation favoured by the analytic situation will under no circumstances be calmed by means of interpretations of the symbolic content, the very excitation of which shows that its meaning has been evacuated by the child. Any interpretation of content is therefore useless and may be experienced by the child as a violent intrusion. It is the analyst's task to understand the transference reasons for which the child has recourse to his *principal* means of defence: the evacuation of meaning via motricity.

Such configurations can also be found in the analyses of neurotic adults. Their noisiest manifestations are acting out and somatization, but this evacuation of meaning can also be detected in inhibition and, above all, in obsessive brooding. However, the situation of relative immobility of the adult patient and the generally higher degree of *manifest conscious* anxiety – proportional to the *latent, unconscious* anxiety – will help to circumscribe the duration and limit the frequency of the most acute forms of these phenomena of evacuation.

This is scarcely possible in the child whose capacities for and cathexis of verbal thinking are still limited, and in whom the severity of the superego very often prohibits the manifest expression of anxiety, leaving him with no other solution than turning to forms of motor discharge, facilitated by the situation of play. It is precisely this intermediate situation of play that constitutes, for the psychoanalyst, the terrain of transforming motor discharge and its attendant evacuation of meaning into an attempt to "dramatize" the intrapsychic and interpersonal conflicts of the child.

The first displacement and the nature of the second object: personal hypotheses

Many French authors have concurred with Klein and the English school on the question of the precocity of a triangulation of the child's emotional organization. For instance, René Diatkine and Janine Simon see triangulation as a consequence of the early splitting of the object and insist on the complexity of the object-relations and identifications that are established during the second semester of a baby's psychic life, with the mother and the "non-mother who must also be able to be a substitute for the mother" (Diatkine & Simon, 1972, p. 398). Of course, this second object will initially be experienced as an extension of the first. And yet its very appearance suggests that the baby's psychic life has already undergone sufficient maturational modifications for it to begin to be able to change its first pre-objectal and fusional perception of the world.

We are accustomed in our day-to-day clinical work to directing our attention towards configurations in which relations with the child's first object have not gone well, with the result that the child – or, later, the child in the adult – cathects the second object with all the pre-forms of expectation addressed to the defective first object. Consequently, he will scarcely be able to cathect his epistemophilic impulses in the discovery of something new and different around this second object.

Nevertheless, as the formation of this second object does not take place in the same *psychic time* as that of the first, its psychical history in the infantile organization can never be superimposed on, or reduced to, that of the first object, even if the cathexes of the first object form the basis of its early elaborations. This second birth is governed by infant's painful discovery that he has not been able to conserve permanently the presence of a first object, and further that this object's good aspects have still not been introjected sufficiently to permit the infant to wait for it with confidence when it disappears for too long from the perceptual field. Even though they are fragile, these introjections nonetheless exist and offer a model of meaning that suffices to direct and support the impulse-driven quest for a second object, except in cases of primary autism.

It is thus important to bear in mind that, since the transference is based, strictly speaking, on the psychic mechanism of displacement, it has its origin in the difficult issue of the first object-loss, and thus in the first work of mourning. This mourning of a primary maternal object – an object that had underpinned the omnipotence of "His Majesty the Baby" living in a state of fusion with it according to the principle *pars pro toto* that characterizes the identificatory relationship with any part-object – would quite simply not be conceivable if it did not liberate a portion of the instinctual drive energy that is henceforth made available for a new cathexis. Indeed, it is in the state of despair, rebellion and fear of destroying this loved/hated object that eludes him that the infant discovers the distinct and autonomous existence of a mother whom he had hitherto believed to be part of himself. Now it is precisely out of this depressive crucible that this second object emerges. Just as all the hopes disappointed by the first object will be transposed on to it, so, in my view, will the whole object's characteristic of autonomy which forms part of the very first constellation of the paternal object from the outset.

In other words if it is true, as my day-to-day clinical experience suggests, that as soon as the first outlines of triangulation appear, every human being functions simultaneously and at every age in the double register of part-object relations and whole-object relations, it is equally true that in the infant the respective proportions of each of these modes of relating will differ depending on whether it is the relationship to the mother or the father that is in question. The sexual specificity of the father will be perceived very early on by the infant, a perception that is underpinned by the advent of genital impulses just at the moment when this first difficult issue of object-loss arises.

The father will thus very swiftly be perceived as not-mother/whole object, equipped with a penis/part-object. The latter is both the carrier/representative of the oral impulses as heir of the nipple, and carrier/representative of the genital impulses as the object of a newly discovered mode of relating: the whole object-relationship. On the other hand, recognition of the mother as a whole object, equipped with a vagina/part-object, is much more problematic, and we may ask ourselves whether it ever will be totally recognized. Indeed, real and lasting recognition of the mother as a whole object constitutes an asymptote of psychic development. This is because the vagina is both a carrier/representative of the genital impulses which mark the definitive loss of the fusional relationship with the breast/part object and the carrier/representative of the impulses to return to the womb, a lost and unrepresentable object and the probable locus of the projection of split-off death drives at the moment of the expulsion of birth. Is it not, moreover, in this very place that the so-called unisex sexual theories of the child[1] and the inflationist metapsychological theories of the phallus have their roots?

Furthermore, in my view the foregoing implies that the penis can only be experienced as a part-object owing to a regressive confusion with the nipple or faeces. This regressive path is illustrated by the well-known fantasy of the "phallic mother", a conglomerate that it would be more exact to call the "phallic breast", since it illustrates a regressive compromise occurring after the discovery of the second object. By means of this compromise, the child refuses to accord the first object with the quality of "whole-object-therefore-disappointing"; he regresses to the point of treating it as a part-object, while attributing the nipple with the phallic dimensions and qualities recognized in the father. This he does with the aim of re-establishing a state of narcissistic satisfaction through projective identification with a new re-idealized edition of the primary maternal object.

The myth of the sphinx, a conglomerate of pregenital characteristics calculated to mask the desirable and desiring femininity of the fertilizable woman that the child cannot satisfy, may also be considered from this perspective. He will then turn the mother into a monstrously self-sufficient character as well as a devourer of fresh flesh. Sexual ambiguity as a denial of the difference between the sexes is essential for eliminating:

1 Genital rivalry with the father for possession of the mother.
2 Fraternal jealousy of the contents of the maternal body, confusedly imaged in the condensed form of babies-*in utero*, penis-in-the-vagina and faeces-in the-anus.
3 Devouring envy of the creative sexuality of the parents in the primal scene.

The Oedipus-child will claim, moreover, that this bivalently gendered Sphinx asks terrible and mysterious questions – the same ones, in fact, that he asks himself about the difference between the generations – and that it cruelly devours all those who venture into the territory of the primal scene.

However that may be, what I want to establish is that:

1 Oedipal experience can be found in all children who come for analysis – apart from primary autistic children, concerning whom I do not feel able to formulate an expert opinion.
2 The difficulty and the didactic interest of child analyses lies in the obligation we have of finding the red thread of the transference through a maze of part-object and whole-object relations that are permanently interwoven, superimposed and opposed, in a defensive pregenital

disorder whose reorganization, always uncertain and temporary, we must promote under the primacy of the genital organization.

The analyst as a part-object

The frequent defusion of the libidinal and destructive impulses makes it difficult, moreover, to identify attacks originating in love as compliant submissions that conceal a bomb. Now, from the point of view of our countertransference, we are less likely to recognize part-object relations in our analysands, probably because we scarcely like to be taken for one of these objects, and for good reason. Each time we are experienced as a part-object by an analysand, we will be treated despotically and arrogantly, penetrated in a casual or insidiously intrusive way, manipulated violently and expelled in an offhand manner, with complete scorn for the effect it has on us. Freud had already been impressed by the *belle indifférence* of hysterics, who seem totally unaware of the forms of care that could be bestowed on the loved object other than those related to pleasure. In my view, this indifference is in no way limited to a single nosographical category; however, while "*belle*" in hysterics and perverse in others, it is always the mark of the predominance of a mode of narcissistic part-object relating over a mode of whole-object relating.

It will also be recalled that the part-object is attributed by the subject with unlimited powers commensurate with infantile omnipotence. As such it is held to be responsible for the best and the worst, for Paradise and Hell: the most absolute love, the most ethereal idealization, the most frenetic possessiveness, the most insolent manipulation, the most murderous jealousy, the most insidious forms of intrusiveness, the most pernicious envy, the most crushing scorn, the most ferocious hatred and the most unnameable terror are some of the affects that tie a subject to his part-objects, internal and external – and we are far from always being able to discern, put into words and interpret the dynamics of feelings that are so difficult to accept in ourselves.

And yet we have all lived through and experienced this essentially pre- and paraverbal world. We have feared it, too, due to the instinctual drive intensity which, at this minimal level of ego-organization, constantly undoes the first outlines of our sense of identity. In this context, the primary part-object – the breast – is the only link with ourselves and with the external world, for the best and the worst. Its loss, felt to be irremediable, plunges us into a world without spatial/temporal boundaries captured so well by Lamartine: "Sometimes, only one person is missing and the whole world seems depopulated". Rage and despair, the last bastions against psychic death, will have the double effect of accelerating the disintegration of the link between subject and object, but also of trying to recover it sadistically, cannibalistically (orally), and even murderously (anally) – a process in which it will be difficult to identify the libido, even though it is still present.

Interpretation of defence, defence through interpretation

When our function as adult analysts brings us into contact with aspects of our analysands' minds, the analytic setting allows us to create a "well-tempered couch", to use the felicitous expression of Jean-Luc Donnet (1995). Child analysis leaves us scarcely any modifiable margins; it is the kingdom of "all or nothing":

- *All*, this is in the case of young children or violent adolescents or alternatively with very ill children, where the rise of excitation is impossible to control and the analyst is faced with the diabolic temptation to defend himself by means of vicious pseudo-interpretations reflecting attacks that he is unable to absorb serenely.
- *Nothing*, this is the situation, particularly with children in the latency period, that risks becoming "frozen" in a sort of narcissistic paralysis, with each of the protagonists spying on the other, while simultaneously trying to conceal himself from the other – here we are right in the midst of part-object relating.

What has happened here? How has this insufferable purring taken the place of a living relationship? Why is the analyst unable to reintroduce the Oedipal situation and sexuality into the clinical picture in a dynamic way? In some analysands – child and even adult – there exists an astonishing power to immobilize perception and thinking in the analyst's countertransference in such a way that he persistently feels "simply silly", embarrassed and powerless – in a word, castrated.

This is because our predominant mode of functioning, which aims to establish links and to understand, disrupts that of the child in latency, whether it is a child who, on account of his age, is actually in the latency period or an adult who, quite clearly, has a child-in-latency within his infantile neurosis. There exists, in any case, a natural discrepancy between the structure and the qualities of the internal psychic space of the adult, on the one hand, and of the child on the other: the first is solidly organized around secondary repression, whereas the second presents a heteroclite structuring that is evolving. This entails consequences for the organization and preservation of the setting, internal and external, in child analysis, for if the excitation of the young child risks overwhelming the analyst's containing capacities, he will undoubtedly find himself more silently disturbed by the child in the period of latency, whose biggest concern is to separate, by means both of repression and splitting, affects from ideational

material related to sexuality. The immediate benefit from this way of proceeding is that of keeping intact a non-sexual idealized image, and often, even a non-gendered image of the world of adults. The secondary benefit, much more subtle and hidden, is that of maintaining in the adult's eyes the image of a child who is not interested in sexuality so as to be able to continue to observe the adult's sexuality without being unmasked.

If we succeed, then, in analysing our countertransference, we will discover that we have at least partially entered into collusion with the omnipotent narcissism of the analysand who seeks to paralyze the primal scene and the impulses that it might arouse in him. He thus stimulates our own narcissistic omnipotence which is only too happy to use this opportunity to get rid of our troublesome infantile sexuality that is excited by the primal scene represented by the analytic relationship. Here we are touching on the problems of the erotization of thought and intellectual inhibition in the analyst.

Classically, a reflection of this transference/countertransference narcissistic collusion can be found in the misrecognition by the therapist of the infantile sexuality expressed in the games and drawings of children. This leads him, when the sexual valency of the material becomes far too evident, and in his efforts to counter-cathect it, to offer the child tautological pseudo-interpretations concerning the contents represented (primal scene, masturbation, etc.) instead of focusing attention on the affect representing them (shame, vengeance, terror, etc.). The analyst's sexual excitation will enter into collusion with that of the patient and, if this patient is a child, he will go on the rampage and make a mess of the therapy room; if, that is, he does not refuse from thereon to come to his sessions.

Genital impulses and epistemophilic impulses

More subtly, this type of countertransference may sometimes make the analyst forget that it is in the psychoanalytic order of things that the child, like the adult, forms his transference neurosis around fixation points that cause him problems and bring into play the compulsion to repeat. Consequently, in both, but more so in the child on account of his genital apragmatism, it is natural that the genital impulses mark time in the transference process at the beginning of the analytic treatment.

On the other hand, it is absolutely certain that the question of the epistemophilic impulses occupies the foreground for the child in analysis. The more we are dealing with younger patients or more immature patients, the more we must expect in analysis to be faced often and intensely with transference issues concerning desire and the danger of knowing. In the child, who is both sexually and psychically immature, as well as physically and psychically dependent on his object of love and hate, the urge to know and its counter-cathexis, intellectual inhibition, will be at the basis of the establishment of the transference/countertransference relationship and will modulate all the vicissitudes of the expression of infantile sexuality.

This configuration will encourage the analyst to relativize the significance of certain transference expressions, arising directly from the period of asking "why?" in children of around the age of 3, whose intrusive nature or arrogance may astonish or shock him. The counterpart of this almost brutal – in its direct aggression or in its obtuse inhibition – manner of being addressed, which he will sometimes simply have to tolerate, will be discovered in the pleasure that he has of gaining access much more quickly and easily, generally speaking, to communication with the child's psychic reality than to that of the adult, whose defences are older and more structured, particularly in an obsessional mode of reifying emotional phenomena.

Analytic listening and therapeutic process

Authentic listening on the analyst's part is perceived immediately by the child, who is so accustomed to being perceived and considered only in the light of his actions, which are merely the reflection of the infantile projections of the adults around him. An 11-year-old girl who was asked by the analyst at the end of the first interview if she wanted to come back to see her replied: *"Oh, yes! No one has ever listened to me like that before!"* It is this rare and precious recognition of the child's psychic reality by the adult that favours the immediate establishment of a basic transference, whose elements will organize themselves and be explored according to the dynamic characteristic of the unfolding of every analytic process. Let us recall that Meltzer (1967) regards the description of the analytic process of the child as the prototype of the psychoanalytic process – given equal conditions, of course, regarding the *frequency of sessions, attention, and interpretative activity* on the part of the analyst.

The passive splitting of the child's psychic reality

Without speaking of massive organic disorders, in particular neurological disorders, or of primary autism, it is important to note that most of the obstacles that prevent the healthy establishment of psychic reality in the child are in the order of trauma, and of very early and more or less prolonged disturbances of parental psychic functioning: either the child has suffered losses or early separations, repeated or prolonged, from his parents, or they have been physically present but psychically absent, denying consciously or unconsciously the existence of psychical qualities in the infant.

The child's psychic life will then be subject to *passive splitting* which will have diverse consequences depending on the parental pathology and on the instinctual drive potentialities of the infant. We must always bear in mind, however, that this splitting will result in an extremely important level of unconscious guilt in the child, guilt about possessing a psychic or even physical life that belongs to him, while it is denied by his internal parents, in particular by his internal mother, his first object.

A diversified pathology of the processes of introjection may then be observed. They can:

1 Be blocked by a massive defence as in secondary autism.
2 Take place anarchically as in infantile psychoses.
3 Give rise to confusional states owing to an inadequacy of active splitting.

On the contrary, the infant may be led to introject massively a maternal depressive state denied by the mother herself and by those immediately around her, obliging him to put all his emerging psychic capacities in the service of an uninterrupted and desperate effort to manically repair a mind that is not his own. In the same vein, he may find he is alone in trying to give meaning to early traumas unrecognized as such by those around him. In all these scenarios, when the child later presents himself to the analyst, he will carefully conceal the essential aspects of his psychic life which has hitherto been nothing but the cause of anxieties that may even include terror and depersonalization. The schizoid mechanisms of excessive splitting and pathological projective identification described by Klein (1946) will then occupy the foreground, unless melancholic depression, which is not as rare in the child as is often thought, has set in insidiously, concealing itself by all means possible from the analyst's interest and concern.

A clinical example

A physiologically prepubescent 12-year-old boy was hospitalized after attempting to commit suicide: he had swallowed some pills just after his mother had gone out to do the shopping; immediately plunged into a state of panic by what he had done, he went to warn his father who was playing in the garden with his brothers.

When he was brought to the consultation by his parents, the analyst asked him to draw his family: he drew two boys of roughly the same size, well-built and with plenty of details. "They are my brothers", he said. In reality they were aged 15 and 8 respectively. He then sketched a face which he crossed out; then the head, the neck and one of the arms of a girl. He then stopped drawing this character and said: "My sister". In reality, this sister was 18 years old. She was the oldest of the siblings. Then he turned the sheet of paper round 180 degrees and drew:

- *His father*, with a nice hat on his head, holding a sickle in one hand and a hammer in the other.
- *His mother*, holding a book in one hand and a lady's handbag in the other. She was dressed in trousers and high-heeled shoes to which he added wheels because, he said: "I didn't manage to draw the tips of the shoes touching the ground and without them she was in danger of falling". A lead was attached to his mother's belt, on the end of which, between father and mother, was a baby with huge ears: "The baby", he said, though in reality the youngest child in the family was his 8-year-old brother.

Then he gave some coherence to this drawing in which the characters are arranged "head- to-tail" by means of what could be considered as the equivalent of a rationalization: he drew a zigzagged line that began under the feet of the father/mother/baby trio, made a curve to form a little hollow space in which he drew water and a tiny round-shaped fish, all of which was topped by a little bridge. The line continued, forming a second hollow, then a third one under the brothers' heads, who thus looked as if they had fallen out of the sky. He signed the whole thing by drawing a sign on which one could read: "Beware: Martians falling".

The first drawing of this intelligent child, whose non-psychotic structure was confirmed thereafter, expresses the inner drama that led him to want to do away with himself – the conscious motivation being a bad note at school, without consequences for his future, and for which he knew that his parents would not reprimand him excessively.

But where is he in the drawing? Well, precisely, he is suppressed both as a person and as a subject conscious of his identity. But although he does not exist as a 12-year-old boy, as part of the sibling group, he is not however absent from the drawing: he is the crossed-out face, without eyes or ears, with no voice, nose, body or genitals. He is the baby listening to everything being said between mummy and daddy, while at the same time he is attached to his mother like a loving and faithful little dog. This mother who has many attributes – men's trousers and a lady's handbag, a baby-little dog and a book, all attributes of bisexuality, knowledge and creativity, so to speak – seems herself to find it difficult to keep her feet on the ground. Fortunately, her humoristic son has provided her with wheels to help her go more quickly, unless, that is, it is because he wants to see her sprawled out on the ground. The analyst will be well-advised to keep this question in mind for the rest of the therapy. As for the father, he is apparently very virile, rather monolithic, less ambiguous and at the same time less subtle: he builds with one hand and castrates with the other, drawing on a group mentality which has a proven track record in the efficacy of psychological intoxication, denunciation and ideological repression. The analyst will have to be more cautious when offering interpretations. This opening on to the *socius* also provides an illustration of my hypothesis concerning the quality of whole object with which the father, in my view, is invested at the outset, making him above all a guarantor of external reality, whereas the mother retains, alongside her quality of whole object, many attributes attesting to the permanence of part-object relations. Moreover, it was her momentary and announced absence alone that caused the child's anxious and suicidal *raptus*.

If we pursue our enquiry into the presence of the drawer in the drawing, we can find him again in the little fish *in utero*, identified with the little brother whose birth eight years earlier caused him pain that he has not forgotten. We also find him identified projectively with the well-built brothers – who will "*tomber des nues*" (*lit.* "fall from the clouds"; *fig.* be stunned) on learning of his tragic exploit –, that is, these Martians who are going to make huge holes in mother-Earth, without being harmed in the slightest way – a manic denial of his castration anxieties. Last but not least, this boy is the author of a drawing who:

1 Ironically places in his father's hands emblems that are far removed from his political, professional and social position.
2 Clearly hopes that his mother who is too complete – thus without desire for him – will fall flat on her face while roller skating with high-heeled shoes.
3 Accuses her of preferring to hold a book in her hand rather than her baby.
4 Shows how the coordinates of the child's world are the exact opposite of those of the adult's world.
5 Comes, nonetheless, up against a central problem, which his sarcastic humour cannot resolve, namely, the difference between the sexes.

Not only is his mother in trousers but, what's more, his sister is not represented below her shoulders and her only arm displays the biceps of a weightlifter! Faced with the pubertal surge of his genital impulses, this 12-year-old boy cannot elaborate his anxieties about being castrated by the father which are normally associated with it. His brothers seem to succeed, he thinks, because they are able to play with the father when the mother goes away; but he cannot. He regresses in an alarming way when faced with this topsy-turvy world and finds no other solution for his love for his mother – love menaced by detachment on account of puberty – than to die.

The parents' transference in the analyst's countertransference

The analysis of adult patients may be described as a situation involving *two generations*: the patient, and the analyst as a support and container of the patient's internal objects, essentially of his very first cathexes of parental objects. The analytic treatment of children, on the other hand, comprises *three generations*: the patient, his parents on whom he depends in more than one respect, but above all affectively, and the analyst, who will therefore become not only the support and the container of the child's internal objects but also, more or less cryptically, that of the internal objects of each of the two parents.

In the light of my clinical experience, I would say that the child analyst must, if the analytic treatment is to proceed smoothly, do everything in his power to establish direct relations with both the patient's parents; and this is true in all circumstances, even when the child is living in an institution or has not seen one of his biological parents for very many years, or since birth. He is, in effect, always cathected transferentially by the parents as the representative of their own parents. I was 24, single, and without children when I discovered this truth/psychic reality which made a big impression on me then and has never dwindled since. The analyst needs to be particularly attentive to his relations with the parents. He must be able to detect both the anxiety and guilt as well as the narcissistic hurt of those who are led to ask for help with their child, thereby recognizing their limits, their suffering related to feelings that they are failing as parents, even if they express this in accusing and projective terms, in particular with regard to the child in question.

Whatever their respective ages are, the parents will project their parental superego into the child analyst. The more severe it is, the more ambivalent they will be. It will be the analyst's task to succeed in unburdening them of this guilt by explaining clearly the role that he expects them to play in a therapeutic alliance which, compared with that which is established in an adult analysis, will thereby have this particularity of involving several people.

He will only be credible insofar as the parents can see that he has a real capacity to identify with their distress and anxiety, a capacity that is linked to great modesty in the face of the suffering inherent in the development of every human being.

The child analyst is the "parent of the parents" at the same time as being the repository of the internal objects created by their personalities in the patient/child he is caring for, and he will need to exercise very close discernment with regard to the analytic space in which he is moving. He will consider the transference of the parents as a valuable gift, a token of the exceptional confidence that they are showing in him by letting him intervene in the most intimate and precious aspect of the child, namely, his psychic life, even – or perhaps especially – if this psychic life has remained an enigma for them and is denied because they deny their own. The child's transference must be received in the same way, but with the aim of being utilized and interpreted, as with any patient in analysis.

The countertransference trap for the analyst consists in the fact that the inner picture that he forms of his patient's parental imagos within the transference/countertransference relationship is intensified by the external perception he has of the real parents of the patient, and by the personal relationship that he has with them. In fact, if his interest for psychic life is what motivates his professional practice, the external aspects of the relationship will only interfere minimally, even if these external aspects are part of his psychic life. Just as this occurs session after session, from one analysand to another, throughout the analyst's working day, so too he has the internal means to recover his capacities for thinking through his personal experience of analysis. If the situation of the analyst working in an institution calls for particular comments that I will make later in this book (see Chapter 12), in all cases there is an infallible means of identifying blockages in the countertransference in child analysis: every time the analyst feels inwardly in conflict with the picture he has of one of the members of the child's entourage, it is very likely that an intrapsychic conflict is involved at the level of his countertransference, probably between his parental imagos and his own Infantile (see Chapter 1).

Note

1 See Chapter 2.

Chapter 10

On the women of *Don Giovanni*

Some aspects of female auto-erotism

> "A woman's body becomes Don Juan's autoerotic double. She is only a part of his body, and vice versa. . . . Nothing about a woman escapes Don Juan, and certainly he 'satisfies' women at their highest level of phallic auto-eroticism".
>
> Jean Gillibert, *De L'auto-eroticisme*, 1977

I have tried, deriving immense pleasure from doing so, to follow one of the innumerable avenues opened up by Jean Gillibert in his exemplary work on the apparently monolithic domain of auto-eroticism.

Don Juan's auto-eroticism requires an object to be accomplished: women. So I tried to understand what made this object so easily accessible to Don Juan. I did this through the fantasies suggested to me by the three female roles created by Mozart – and Da Ponte – in the famous opera *Don Giovanni* (K527) of 1787.

What are the narcissistic and instinctual drive structures in women upon which Don Juan characteristically has such an immediate and total impact? For even if Leporello – the "lower part of Don Juan" as Pierre-Jean Jouve calls it, and which could well be Don Juan's ego, an ego that is weak and reduced to slavery by its perverse impulses – exaggerates in the aria *mille e tre*, it seems to me essential to the coherence of the myth of Don Juan to admit that he has real success with women and that he satisfies them, in a certain way.

According to Brigitte and Jean Massin, Don Juan lives for the moment, while Evelyne Kestemberg considers him as a teenager. And it is a fact that the juvenile trepidation of his extraordinary vitality, unhampered by any obsessional doubt or even by time for reflection, can make him the typical embodiment of manic phallic splendour. In addition, Don Juan knows how to speak to women. Thanks, perhaps, to a projective identification with his own female side which he tolerates better when it is projected than introjected, he always manages intuitively to find the right angle in fantasy from which his partner wishes to be wooed. In other words, for each of them he finds the precise point of impact on the narcissistic roots of their mode of object-relating:

1 In Donna Anna, pride in being the object of a passion that can include rape, and even murder.
2 In Zerlina, the enchantment of the little girl who suddenly sees herself becoming the heroine of a fairy tale, a shepherdess loved by Prince Charming – the father's ideal penis.
3 In Donna Elvire, finally, the hoped-for satisfaction of having found the "man of her life", the companion, the one with whom she would like to have a child.

But Don Juan is always fleeing. For him it is about exerting sadistic anal control over an object-relationship, the large part of which he feels eludes him. It is also about the orgastic escalation of his greedy orality and his compulsion to tirelessly challenge at a phallic level his terror of what he sees in the female as an absence of sexual organs. Always on the lookout for his own female side – which he dreads because it is condensed with his castration anxieties and contains his oral greed and anal sadism – Don Juan also flees thanks to this feminine double, his own internal psychic space. Each woman is the receptacle of the affects and object relationships that irresistibly attract him, but for which he never manages to take responsibility himself. It is for this reason that he masters the arts of arousing, exciting and bringing to their peak women's desires and emotions, which are possible but necessarily distorting mirrors of what he expects yet refuses to experience in himself.

Brief encounters with oneself

It is therefore incumbent on Don Juan's women to express the whole array of object relationships that he seeks and rejects, almost simultaneously, in his brief encounter with each of them, only to find himself ever more dramatically locked into his repetitive auto-eroticism. Each of the three female roles in *Don Giovanni* seemed to me to show, moreover, one of the points of fixation and one of the modes of regression on which Don Juan can make a woman stumble. These are obviously only three possibilities among many others, since it is precisely at the level of the complexity of his desire and his object-relating that Don Juan seems to me to hurt woman most deeply. Indeed, Don Juan reveals a woman to herself, including her genital impulses, yet it is with voyeuristic passion and with the aim of better denying the importance of this discovery, while retreating to his position of systematic withdrawal: the negation of the difference of the sexes, the reduction of the other to the same, that is to say, in the image of what happens in a cancerous tissue: dedifferentiation. It is, therefore, a regressive dedifferentiation of the genital sphere into the pregenital sphere, of the whole object-relationship into a part-object relationship, of introjective identification into a range of other identifications, including projective or narcissistic identification, mimetic or adhesive projection, and maybe imagoic too.

Donna Anna chooses an Oedipal rival in Ottavio who in no way overshadows the prestigious lustre of her father, the Commander. This choice takes into account the difference of the generations – the young Ottavio has his whole life ahead of him in which to prove himself. However, the choice of the range of the role (tenor) – classical but not binding from the strict point of view of the "opera" form – the very asexual alliance that is established between him and Donna Anna and, finally, the repeated avoidance by Ottavio of confrontation with Don Juan, all suggest that the difference of the sexes is not really incorporated into Donna Anna's choice. It is Don Juan, heir to the sexual father, who reveals this difference to her, and in an overwhelming, cataclysmic way. But he goes on to deny it a moment later, treating, if we are to believe the superb vocal intensity of the role of Donna Anna, what was indeed, for her, the discovery of orgasm, as a child's game. Don Juan flees at this very moment, leaving her alone to face an unintegratable experience of her newly discovered femininity. She then also regresses to a phallic position, that is to say she decathects her vagina, abandoned by the penis. She literally runs after the penis as if it were her own sexual organ, and this is when she exclaims: "*No sperar, se non m'uccidi, ch'io te lascia fuggir mai!*" ("There's no hope, unless you kill me, that I'll ever let you go!").

Metaphorically, the death of the Commander represents the collapse of all Donna Anna's phallic identifications, and particularly their superego and ego ideal aspects. Moreover, as she is the only one of the three women to be devoid of any maternal image – Donna Elvira has her handmaiden, who, moreover, is courted by Don Juan, and Zerlina has Donna Elvira and all the young girls at her wedding – Donna Anna will definitely not be able to integrate her femininity. So we see her wandering until the end of the drama, torn between the vengeance she demands against Don Juan and the vivid memory of their momentary intimacy. Her words, "I'm dying!" are authentic: they express both the "little death" (of ecstasy) through identification with a rival who is experiencing it, and the death of her bisexuality.

It goes without saying that this brings us back to the difficulty, in such women, of mourning a first object, narcissistically the bearer of all goodness, whose displacement onto a second object, the penis, often leaves in its wake much unsatisfied oral greed, even bound up with envy, which will spoil their relationship with men. It is precisely here that Don Juan is able to make his impact on them, presenting himself, by virtue of his brilliance, as being able to satisfy everything. It is striking to see that Donna

Anna denies any compensatory role for Ottavio who demands it explicitly, while continuing to hound Don Juan as if he were the only one who could settle this account. He, at least, is the only one to claim to be able to do so, for seduction, even if phallic, always refers to a part-object relationship where the boundaries between the different elements of the penis-faeces-baby-nipple equation are blurred.

Zerlina, from a sociohistorical point of view, represents ancillary love affairs, with all that they induce in the way of indulgence towards the small child: any mother can smile serenely at her little daughter who, at around three years, declares: "When I grow up, I will marry Daddy!" On the other hand, she will be more worried when this same child, having become a beautiful teenager, agrees without hesitation to be wooed by an old fop.

The Zerlina-Don Juan duet – *"Laci darem la mano. . . . Vorrei e non vorrei"* ("There you will give me your hand. . . . I'd like to, but yet I would not".) – has the same freshness as the Cherubino aria in the *Marriage of Figaro*, the child, Eros. We are caught up and charmed by these games whose candid appearance and "auto-erotic" impact mask the brazen effrontery involved, for which Masetto pays the price. At the same time as it protects her from Don Juan's perversity, Zerlina's polymorphism fits in perfectly with it. She hardly seems to suffer from having been seduced by Don Juan, as if genitality still had for her only the reduced place it has in children's sexual games. Just enough to make it possible to "behave like grown-ups", this cumbersome genitality is then split-off and re-projected on to the maternal image – in this case, Donna Elvira – allowing Zerlina to reappear asking her husband to beat her; for it is undoubtedly true that the conventional pregenitality of sadomasochistic relationships makes them by far the simplest and most solid, and devoid of any soul-searching.

Donna Elvira, on the other hand, is the woman who suffers most directly from her relationship with Don Juan because she is the only one who really loves the person of Don Juan, even if she also exudes her laments, her bitterness and her narcissistic wounds. In support of this statement, I will make two arguments:

1 The fact that Mozart used the theme of Glück's Orpheus, "I have lost my Eurydice", for Elvira's first lament.
2 The attitude of Donna Elvira who, at the end of the second act, attempts the impossible to save Don Juan, without letting herself be stopped by the stinging humiliations that he inflicts on her by aping her hopeless love.

It is left to her to cry for Eurydice, a female double, both of herself and Don Juan, who is doubly struck with inertia before being engulfed in the hell of persecution, ignorance and sterility of compulsive repetition. She becomes the receptacle for all the tears that Don Juan has never been able to shed, all the affects he has been unable to experience, and all the fantasies that he has repressed, trapped as he is in fascination and horror of his own internal psychic space, which he experiences too directly as his female side filled with hidden desires.

Auto-eroticism, castration and identifications

These brief considerations on the three female characters of Mozart's *Don Giovanni* have allowed me to portray auto-eroticism as the result of a regressive dedifferentiation of the object relationship. Thus auto-eroticism can manifest itself at each stage of development, especially on the occasion of the important events that mark human existence: adolescence, engagement, break-ups, marriage, maternity and paternity, the departure of children who have become adults, middle-age crisis, etc., without forgetting the explosive field of professional success and failure.

I therefore concur with Jean Gillibert when he suggests that Don Juan "'satisfies' women at their highest level of phallic auto-eroticism", provided that this auto-erotic phase is considered as a second phase, a regressive phase of reorganization of an intense experience that is forever lost, with all its attendant Oedipal echoes. Furthermore, I think that there are other levels of regressive reorganization, where auto-eroticism always appears as a sign of the deterioration of the relational fabric, generally around the essential core of the personality. If we use the metaphor proposed by *Don Giovanni* one last time, this nucleus could be:

1 For Zerlina, around what Freud (1923b) designated as "the infantile genital organization" between the ages of 3 and 4.
2 For Donna Anna, at the post-pubertal stage of the reshaping the genital impulses, which must permanently move away from parental imagos and be invested in partners of the subject's own generation.
3 For Donna Elvira, finally, at the subtle and complicated point of impact of the maternal sphere on female genitality.

Perhaps Don Juan is always experiencing the same thing. At least he seems fiercely determined to do so, and we cannot fail to suspect that he is thereby seeking to deny the castration and death anxieties inherent in the human condition. But by managing to interfere as he does in the narcissistic pole of women whose psychic structures are none the less very different, he seeks to experience what he makes these women experience, and his failure confronts us with the tragic inability to move on from mimetic identification to a more introjective identification, from an "as if" relationship to an authentic object relationship, and to leave repetition behind in favour of creativity. For sneering is never far away, and this is what makes the most tender and passionate movements of Don Juan grate. And if the trombones at the end of the opera give a pompously funereal tone to the erect and petrified sexual member that is the statue of the Commander, it is because we have to mock the love of the parents one last time, to which we owe our very existence, from the moment when, for want of having been able to accept the primal scene, we are definitively caught up, like Don Juan, in the conjunction of castration and death.

Chapter 11

Between the tree and the bark

The psychotherapist in institutions*

The bark

It is often repeated that splits in institutions must be reduced. However, to achieve this aim – one, moreover, that I fully approve of – it is a matter, above all of identifying these splits and of evaluating their quality. Some are adequate and others are not, owing to their functional role and their irreversibility. A human being who did not have a mechanism of splitting would live in a total state of mental confusion: it is therefore a necessary mechanism for all individual psychic organization. But as soon as we dwell on institutional problems, the question of the impact on institutional functioning of this mechanism of splitting that is characteristic of the organization of every individual – whether patient or carer – takes on a different perspective.

Let us begin by examining the classical organization of an institution with therapeutic aims, and we will see that it always has two heads: the medical director and the administrative director. This implies that all the individuals living or working in this place will identify one another in terms of a dual hierarchy: medico-social and administrative. The particularity of this unavoidable dual obedience is one of the factors that favours the mechanism of splitting in each person.

Anyone who has lived or worked in an institutional structure of this kind will have noticed the particularities of the constraints that this dual obedience imposes, especially the inevitable paradoxes linked to the "dual cap" of each of the carers concerning the efficacy of the respective powers and duties attributed to them. These powers and duties which, theoretically, are combined, are in practice oriented and driven by inevitably heterogeneous motivations since they are linked to different hierarchies that supersede them.

The situation of the psychotherapist

To the extent that there are still psychotherapists working in institutions today, it is possible to observe among them several splits relating to their training on the one hand and their place in the institution on the other.

Some psychotherapists who belong, for instance, to the medical profession, are in the institution to complete their professional curriculum by doing an internship placement in psychiatry. If they decide thereafter to pursue a hospital career in the shorter or longer term, they will work their way up through the ranks of the hierarchy of the medical order which includes psychotherapy as a therapeutic act on the same level as an act of prescribing medication. Their identity as a psychotherapist will be derived from the medical studies that they have undertaken, and their nosography will be related to their specialization in psychiatry. They will have few problems in organizing their professional space within the institution, as the administrative hierarchy has long been used to taking into account representatives of the medical hierarchy. Their commitment to psychotherapeutic activity will be of variable duration and geometry, ranging from the internship placement to the post of medical director, according to a well-defined staggering of administrative responsibilities and fees. The role played by the psychotherapeutic function will vary according the taste, gifts, capacities and emotional investments of each of them. For even if his medical director is strongly in favour of psychoanalysis, a young doctor always retains the possibility of modifying his orientation by moving to another department or institution, without losing his socio-professional identity as a specialist doctor in so doing.

Thus, the external aspects of the phenomena of transference will be familiar to the young intern in psychiatry insofar as he will be able to link them to the power attributed to his medical knowledge by the caregiving team and by the patients. The unconscious determinants of the transference will, however, remain foreign and obscure to him until he has successfully completed a real training in psychotherapy, a more personal than professional training one might say, the prototype of which remains personal psychoanalytic experience. In effect, it is only the latter that teaches us to observe and discover from the inside some of the parameters forming the infinite complexity of the mode of functioning of the ego and of internal psychic objects, as well as their interrelations with the objects and persons of the external world.

Other psychotherapists working in institutions have had a university training in clinical psychology. They have done a minimum of five or six years of university studies and possess either a vocational master's degree, a research master's degree or a doctorate in psychology. They have been trained to observe painstakingly the intellectual, psycho-sensory, psychomotor and affective manifestations of the individuals they are investigating, and very severely cautioned against anything that might resemble diagnostic or therapeutic activity, which would expose them to accusations of practising medicine illegally. However, since the 1960s, prestigious leading figures in psychiatry have deemed it useful to join forces with psychologists in their research work, in establishing their diagnoses, and in the conduct of their therapies. The psychologist/psychotherapist thus finds himself in the same situation as the doctor/psychotherapist concerning the obligation to undertake a second training if he wants to fulfil his functions, that is to say a personal psychoanalytic experience.

And yet, while this personal experience helps him to improve his efficiency in the institution considerably, it does not, however, constitute an opening at the level of his socio-professional evolution. Indeed, for reasons that stem from the history of his profession – in particular, the fact that he has chosen to retain the status of liberal profession – the psychologist today does not belong to the category of medical auxiliaries. As, moreover, psychoanalytic scientific societies remain hesitant to establish themselves as a professional order, the administrative hierarchy of institutions can only offer the psychologist/psychotherapist an "uneasy compromise", practically equivalent to that of medical auxiliaries, even if he is a training member of the International Psychoanalytic Association. In other words, his hopes of promotion are almost non-existent, both with regard to his range of remuneration and to his powers of decision-making within the caregiving team. Thus, owing to this double bind, the psychologist/psychotherapist who has done a long personal analysis and successfully accomplished a psychoanalytic training recognized by one or several national and/or international scientific societies constitutes the quintessence of the hybrid in the institution, since he belongs to a doubly non-existent species, in the medical hierarchy and in the administrative hierarchy alike.

I propose to consider this "strange bird" as the *essential* model of the identity of the psychotherapist in institutions. Without power and without membership of a recognized social body, he is required to situate himself in the only position that every psychotherapist, whether doctor/psychiatrist or psychologist, should adopt, and to accept that his only real status is in the psychic life of his patients.

The tree

Now that I have characterized what I consider to be the *social and administrative bark*, I will move on to the description of the tree, that is to say of the life that animates an institution, life with which the psychotherapist – doctor or psychologist – interacts on a daily basis.

When a new psychotherapist is introduced into an institution, the different members of the caregiving team will have a very characteristic range of complex feelings towards him. They will frequently attempt to form a picture of him in advance by finding out whether he is a doctor or a psychologist. In both cases, there is an error of attribution. And if the therapeutic dimension is maintained in the first case, the dimension of knowledge of psychic life is obliterated in both denominations. Furthermore, the doctor is anticipated in fantasy by the team as a paternal image – even in the case of a woman – whereas the psychologist is fantasized in a maternal role, even in the case of a man. In all cases, once the therapist has assumed his functions, the more the population treated in an institution is pathological, the more the discouragement, or even despair, of the other members of the caregiving team will tend to be addressed to the psychotherapist. Given the fantasized configuration that I have just mentioned, significant differences can be observed in the expectations that will be expressed unconsciously towards the psychotherapist/doctor and the psychotherapist/psychologist.

A few examples will help us to look more closely at this situation and to examine the elements of psychic bisexuality in it which, for the caregiving team, set up a very particular fantasized primal scene. The characteristic features of this scene are first and foremost linked to the unconscious place that the therapist has in the group, while they are exogenous to the psychic structure of the patient taken into therapy. This situation, which is specific to working in institutions, resides in the fact that the caregiving team projects on to the patient/therapist couple a primal scene fantasy that interferes with the intimacy of the therapeutic relationship woven between the therapist and his patient, and possibly also with the patient's family. In a way that is apparently perfectly adequate, the dual therapeutic relationship is perceived by the caregiving team as a very primitive mode of feeding and maternal care provided for the undeveloped parts of the patient. The problem arises from the fact that this perception, which is adequate on the conscious level, is accompanied, on the unconscious level, by affects of rivalry and envy, not only in other patients but also in the whole caregiving team. Now every dual therapeutic relationship in an institution is heading for serious trouble if it is not contained and protected by a third party who plays, as it were, a paternal role with regard to the mother/infant dyad. Theoretically, it is for the caregiving team to assume this role. In practice, the conjunction of these two fantasy configurations just outlined makes things much more complicated. Here are a few examples.

A young psychologist/psychoanalyst took a little 5-year-old girl into treatment within the framework of a Medico-Psycho-Pedagogical Centre (CMPP). The parents, who, on the face of it, were very cooperative owing to their child's massive difficulties, agreed to organize for the child to be accompanied there twice a week. The psychotherapy followed its course satisfactorily: the child developed rapidly, and particularly at the level of language. As soon as she overcame her language confusion, the parents found endless pretexts to make her miss her sessions while continuing to repeat hypocritically: "Psychotherapy is indispensable for our child". In spite of his insistence, the psychotherapist could not get the better of this double game based on an envious component on the parents' part concerning the development of their child and the pleasure that she showed in coming to her sessions. Due to classical guilt feelings in young children, the little girl did not feel capable of insisting on having her sessions and the situation was near its breaking-point. The child began once again to experience difficulties in adapting to school, which were then attributed to the psychotherapist's shortcomings. He began to feel very guilty and depressed. He asked himself whether he was feeling too much rivalry with the mother in his countertransference or whether there were elements of transference erotization to which he had not been sufficiently attentive; or alternatively whether he had not misinterpreted the Oedipal situation . . . in short, he was presenting all the symptoms of a depressed mother. Finally, it emerged in supervision that this psychologist/psychoanalyst had great difficulty in securing the interest and cooperation of his head doctor – a woman – for the analytic work that he was the only one, it should be stressed, to provide in this institution. Thanks to the support of the supervision group, he was nonetheless able to set up a meeting between the parents, the head doctor and himself. During this meeting, the psychotherapist felt, for the first time, that he had really been heard by the parents and was able to explain that a therapist is not endowed with supernatural powers – with those, precisely, that the infant attributes in fantasy to his mother – and that analytic therapy is a matter of patient attention to psychic processes and requires regularity that is akin to maternal care. The head doctor, who was herself in analysis, became aware of how she had been avoiding taking on the protective role that she should have played because of the unconscious ambivalence she experienced towards the work of the psychologist/psychoanalyst. It scarcely needs adding that, owing to the un-analysed ambivalence of the parents and to the late change in attitude of the head doctor, the child and the psychotherapist were only able to do three months of regular work before the situation deteriorated once again. My experience leads me to think that it was already an exceptional achievement, given the power of the mechanisms of splitting separating the weak and infantile parts of an individual from their source of development.

Splitting between institutional power and therapeutic activity

When one of the members of the immediate environment of a patient who is having psychotherapy in an institution presents a severe psychopathology, the splitting between the therapeutic tree and the administrative bark will be accentuated in the institution in terms of the way the patient is considered by everyone else. And, as one would expect, it is at the level of individual psychotherapy that splitting between the paternal (institutional power) and maternal (individual psychotherapy) elements will be felt most intensely and lastingly, and will cause the most damage. The characteristics of this splitting may therefore be considered as the health bulletin of the institution. What I mean by that is that for a psychologist/ psychoanalyst who is used to managing his countertransference towards his patients, and their parents if the patient is a child, it is the additional degree of psychic suffering that he feels that will be the measure of the efficiency of the whole institutional therapeutic approach of which he is an integral part. Two illustrations will serve to back up my remarks.

The young girl with unrecognized suffering

In the context of a day hospital, an experienced psychotherapist was doing psychoanalytic psychotherapy with a little girl on a thrice-weekly basis. This child had lost her mother at the age of 2 or 3 and was living with her father and his new wife who could not tolerate her little step-daughter, hit her and tortured her at the level of feeding. Following a court order, the child was removed from her family and placed in this institution and in a foster home. While the psychotherapy was evolving positively, the socio-judicial authorities decided to try to reintegrate this child in her family setting for nights and weekends. Soon enough, the psychotherapist saw the child arriving for her sessions with bruises and abrasions, while she frequently missed school on Mondays and sometimes on other days of the week on various pretexts, but always for short periods of time that did not require the family to produce a medical certificate. The educator and the school teacher also noticed the state the child was in, but the child stuck obstinately to the same version: "I banged myself against a piece of furniture . . . it was the cat that scratched me". In her sessions she became extremely inhibited again or talked falsely in a way that was characteristic of a manic defence. Feeling increasingly anxious and essentially bearing the guilt for this situation alone, the psychotherapist finally managed, after several weeks of insistent requests, to get the head doctor of her institution to personally notice the child's bruises and injuries and to inform the social and judicial agencies about this situation. They took note of the declaration by the day hospital, but decided to leave the little girl in her family setting so as not to "traumatize" the stepmother who, in the meantime, had had a baby! As the management of the day hospital had decided not to take the matter any further either – even though no arrangements had been made to help this stepmother and her baby – the psychotherapist had no other recourse than to scupper herself by announcing that she was stopping the psychotherapy. She explained to the child that it was clear to her that she was being beaten again and that she felt powerless to do anything about it; however, she did not want to collude with what was going on by pretending that she could genuinely analyse her desires and guilt towards internal objects whose external representatives were so deviant. Terrified of those who were mistreating her, this child was obviously not going to denounce them but she finally acquiesced with what the psychotherapist had told her. She even expressed the wish to see the psychotherapist again "when she was older".

Having putting up with the virtuous indignation of the head of the institution as well as of some of her colleagues and representatives of the social-judicial services, this psychotherapist nonetheless had the satisfaction of seeing her courage rewarded: her attitude had seemed sufficiently shocking for the authorities concerned that they agreed to reconsider the situation, resulting in a new placement for the child.

If this situation of being powerless was transformed *in extremis* into one of having power, it was only because the psychotherapist was able to recognize the hidden psychic suffering of this little girl, rather than taking refuge in a so-called "benevolent neutrality" that would have concealed her real powerlessness behind a fantasy of omnipotence. Eléonare Faucher's 2018 film *La maladroite*, based on a true story with a fatal outcome, offers a remarkable portrayal of the obstinately reparative behaviour of battered children and the social and psychological malaise that inhibits the swiftness and efficiency of the intervention of institutions.

The child who was forgotten

A young psychotherapist came to see me one day and said:

> I would like to speak to you about this young boy, because he's the only child in the institution I never think about outside the sessions. When I attend team meetings, I always forget his file (she later forgot it in my office at the end of the supervision!) and I have never managed to give him more than one session a week, even though I have done so with others. I think it is because this child really hurts me psychically.

This 11-year-old child had suffered from severe depressive episodes with attendant delusion formations. His parents were separated and the children had lived for several years in a foster institution. His mother suffered from a mental illness and spent part of her time in a psychiatric hospital and the other in a little maid's room at her parents', where she lived reclusively. Even though she tried to care for her children as best she could when her condition allowed her to exercise her visiting rights, a consensus was imperceptibly reached in the institution that they should only take the father into account, a very communicative person who had no qualms about insisting on the mother's pathology and on his own devotion to the children. He had apparently made a good impression on the social authorities because they had recently returned his children to him by virtue of the fact that he had got remarried. In fact, it turned out that this second wife assumed responsibility alone for the material and psychological welfare of the children and threatened to leave if the father, a smooth talker, did not get a bit more involved in reality.

The psychotherapist had insisted on speaking with the mother one day when she was accompanying her son: "When I saw her", she told me,

> the contact between us was good but I was struck by her painful attitude of helplessness and passivity towards her child. Above all I recognized myself in this helplessness and suffering. It's exactly what I feel in my countertransference towards this young patient.

An analysis of the session material confirmed that in the transference the child was only able to express his relationship of phobic avoidance towards a destroyed and helpless mother, splitting off the rest of his object-relations and identifications – in particular, paternal – in order to withdraw them from analytic investigation in the same way as the father avoided having a real relationship with his son. I encouraged her to try to get her institution to agree to offer the child a second session. This was accepted and supported without difficulty by the excellent team of the CMPP as a whole. To her great surprise, the psychotherapist discovered a child who was extremely eager to understand what was going on in his psychic life, spontaneously and regularly linking up the present session with the one before and, at the end of each session, saying to his psychotherapist: "Please write down on this piece of paper what I would like to understand next time, in case I forget!" In fact, he never forgot. The two parental objects appeared in the transference, as well as the need to distinguish between true and false, provided the child did not feel alone and crushed by depression. The delusional elements disappeared, as they were no longer needed to compensate for feelings of despair that had become intolerable since it was now shared and blended with hope. Last but not least, the therapist no longer suffered, in spite of the very significant technical difficulties raised by this case and, far from forgetting the child or his file, she looked forward to the sessions, as he did, with pleasure and impatience.

The group and the person

I consider that, in an institution, the relationship between the psychotherapist-without decision-making-powers and his patient constitutes *the topological point of the encounter between the private and the social spheres*, that is to say, the meeting-point between the intimacy of the analytic relationship on the one hand and the patient's integration in the group, institution and family on the other.

This relationship between the psychotherapist and his patient occupies a topographical space analogous to that between a mother and her infant, who is a part of herself at the beginning of life but also the fruit of her romance with the father and, consequently, the heir of both their Oedipal configurations and their own identifications. Likewise, the patient in individual psychotherapy is unconsciously experienced by the members of the caregiving team as the fruit of the loves between the mother/psychotherapist and the father/director of the institution – irrespective of the actual genders of the two protagonists.

As the locus for filtering all parasitical projections and at the same time of all future possibilities, the psychotherapeutic relationship derives its force from its very fragility. But it is only possible on the express condition that it is protected and supported by a paternal agency within the institution. If the organization of the caregivers as a whole revolves around this original triad, the consequences of this way of considering individual psychotherapeutic work will make themselves felt in the form of less confusion between the group and the individual and better organization of the splitting that is necessary for the development of each person: there will be better differentiation between internal psychic reality and external reality, and between the inside and the outside of the individual therapeutic relationship. Indeed, we are all familiar with how individual therapies burden the organization of socio-educative groups organized within an institution. It is always just when one is taking one's group for a walk or to the pottery workshop that one remembers that this or that patient has to go for his session of psychotherapy, not to mention other possible clashes with physiotherapy or speech therapy session or with meetings between a patient and his family in the medical consultant's office.

Thus, the more a patient presents pathological splitting – whether active or passive – the more this splitting will have an impact on the institutional, interprofessional and personal splitting of the caregiving team. The triadic organization that I am proposing for the capacity for reverie of each caregiver will hopefully result in a lessening of the pathological dimension of the narcissistic issues involved.

However, while these narcissistic issues concern individuals, I think that they are essentially related to the part of the Self that is governed in each one of us by "group mentality" as studied by Bion after Freud. Now if this group mentality is the element that enables each one of us to try to establish an initial *consensus* with the group to which he belongs, and if, as a result, it may be considered as an initial mode of contact between individuals, it is still the case that it contains within it the danger of the prejudices inherent in any form of functioning that proceeds in the mode of generality.

"Everyone knows very well that . . . , everyone does that . . . , one must never . . . , one must always . . ." are basic verbal expressions of group mentality. In other words, the essence of its areas of consensus is constituted by taboos which, though they form the basis of animal and human socialization, obviously do not take much account of the development of the individual life of the persons who make up the group, and further treat the difference between the sexes and generations from the angle of the preservation of the species and the struggle for the survival of the species. Consequently, the unity of the group will be formed around projecting hate on to the outside – stranger = enemy – and searching for a leader who will be endowed with absolute power in order to make an idol of him.

It is only when a group has functioned and engaged in thought together for a certain period of time in a valid way that respect and interest for the individuality of the persons within the group will be able to develop. But fantasies concerning the primal scene within the group will then come to the fore, while the ideal and the ethic of the group will seek to impose themselves on the relationship of intimacy and the possible exogamy of two individuals. Indeed, the fantasy of the "group-as-genitor" will strive to substitute itself for the reality of the relationship between two people and for the state of parenthood that is immediately associated with it. It is at this last level that a good number of our institutional conflicts are situated, the patient/infant inevitably being experienced, at the unconscious level of the group mentality of each of the members of the team, as the heir of the ideals and taboos of the institutional group, rather than as a human being in his own right. I suggest that this unconscious group ideal be substituted patiently, day after day, by the true ideal that gives us the privilege of working as an institutional team: that of proposing each patient a resumption of his processes of development hindered by the past and illness, in the form of a psychotherapeutic relationship of intimacy with one of the members of the team, a relationship that is protected and supported by one of its other members and considered with benevolent neutrality by the caregivers as a whole.

Note

* In a slightly reorganized form, this text was taken from a communication published in a collective work edited by Gérard Bléandonu et al. (1992) titled *Cadres thérapeutiques et enveloppes psychiques: quatrièmes journées d'étude francophones sur les hôpitaux de jour*.

Chapter 12

Pregenitality and the primal scene, or the phantasized destiny

Of the digestive tract*

Starting from the concept of erogenous zones proposed by Freud (1905) in the *Three Essays on Sexuality*, the study of the phantasized destiny of the digestive orifices of the human body has known various fortunes in psychoanalytic writings, depending on the era and school of thought. While orality has flourished particularly with psychoanalysts of the English School and child psychoanalysts, many French authors have been interested in anality, the pivotal psychic organization between an orality whose archaic and devouring aspects may appear to some as a vulgar affair of a wet-nurse, and a genitality of which the phallus is the undisputed representative. In France, the work of Jean Favreau (Troisier, 1991) Jean Bergeret (1976) and Béla Grunberger (1989) constituted, in their time, fundamental reference points.

I nevertheless think it possible and fruitful to suggest a slightly less fragmented reflection on the image of the subject's own body, a reflection that seeks to connect the various orifices of the digestive tract, considered by Freud as supports for pregenital drive functioning, rather than isolating them on the pretext of a supposed chronology in their respective erogenous polarities. Indeed, as Brusset writes:

> Due to its simplicity, its evocative character, its proximity to direct observation, its immediate references to the body, eroticism and the mother, the Freudian model of libidinal development runs the risk of easy, aberrant, questionable or useless utilizations. . . . So it must remain open, albeit subject to metapsychology and therefore dialectically articulated with the structural point of view.
>
> (Brusset, 1992, p. 121)

In my reflections on the relations of the digestive tract with the fantasy of the primal scene, I will draw mainly on Freud's (1915a) "Instincts and their vicissitudes" as well as on Bion's (1962b) contributions with regard to the first observable instinctual derivatives – which are already very complex – namely, love (L), hate (H) and the urge or desire to know (K). We can see from the start that the question cannot be tackled independently of instinctual drive issues. From the numerous studies of reference devoted to this frontier concept, I would like to mention here the excellent article by Green (1988): "Pulsions, psyché, langage, pensée".

My attempt to study the fantasized organization of the digestive tract does not coincide exactly with the description of the "stages of libidinal development" proposed by Freud (1905) and Abraham (1924) as organizations of the psychic cathexes appearing in a temporal succession inferred from observable behaviour in children.

Many studies have been devoted to what was, in its time, called "genetic psychoanalysis" (Kestemberg & Kestemberg, 1966), and which unleashed the wrath of a large number of French psychoanalysts who denounced, in particular, the trap constituted by the old notion of stages of development, at the frontiers of psychology and psychoanalysis. While joining their criticisms, I do not, however, think that current analytical thinking is totally devoid of implicit references to the stages of libidinal organization as they were described by Freud in the *Three Essays* . . . criticism is easy, but art is difficult. In the course of a thought process, the repressed always returns before one expects it. It is still necessary to distinguish its drive component from its defensive component.

The hypothesis I want to put forward, then, is that the representation of the stages of development eases the intolerable nature of the discovery of infantile sexuality and serves as a defensive formation in the face of its unthinkability. Based on the model of infantile sexual theories, the model of stages therefore constitutes, in my opinion, the defence par excellence against the Freudian discovery of "infantile genital sexuality". The model of the cathexis of the erogenous zones proposed by the theory of stages purely and simply reverses the facts of the problem. By isolating the pregenital zones to place them artificially in "symbolic equation" (Segal, 1957) with the genital apparatus, this model defensively denies *the existence of a cathexis that is already present from the outset and constantly organizing the latter.*

In reality, it is obviously the opposite that occurs, namely a partial de-eroticization of the non-genital zones when psychic development is going well. However, this de-eroticization, the fruit of the work of the *Pcs.*, always remains relative and mobile, depending on the emotional states of moment. It does not damage what I would call the "basic phantasized geography" of the unconscious cathexes of the subject's own body by the libido. All psychopathology, including of course psychosomatics, provides us with evidence of this on a daily basis.

Against this insistence of *genital sexuality* in infants, children and then adults, the anal organization lends itself particularly well to playing the defensive role that one might expect of it; there are two reasons for this:

1 More or less combined with the pregenital phallic organization, it constitutes a phantasized organization of choice against infantile

genitality, which, as has just been recalled, constitutes the most hazardous of Freudian discoveries in this area, because it is the most threatening for the neurotic Oedipal pole in adults.

2 Anality is the only pregenital organization in which the libidinal cathexis is detached from a constrictive relationship with the external object at the level of need.

As a description of an attempt to escape, at least at face value, from the stranglehold of the reality principle by separating it from the pleasure/unpleasure principle, the anal configuration lends itself particularly well to auto-eroticism – but also hypochondria – to idealization – but also paranoia – in short, to many evasions from the reality principle. The problem begins there, moreover, since in my opinion such a disconnection of the two principles of psychic functioning will gradually impoverish one or the other mode of satisfaction: the auto-erotic as well as the relational.

With regard to the fundamental phantasy of the primal scene, whose essential role in Oedipal structuring Freud highlighted in relation to the analysis of the "Wolf Man", the anal organization occupies a pivotal situation making its phantasy content as malleable and reifiable as the physiological content linked to its name. The latter thus often loses any metaphorical and conceptual dimension without, however, giving an accurate account of the sensory and motor valencies of the libidinal cathexes experienced by the subject at the level of his bodily ego (Freud, 1923a; Haag, 2018). However, in examining these valencies more closely, we are led to consider the hypothesis of a very early libidinal cathexis of *the entire digestive tract.*

Of course, this way of looking at libidinal organization does not remove the difficulty inherent in describing the normality of an authentic psychic development. For although it is relatively easy to refute the notion of stages as an organization destined to be surpassed, it is more difficult to sustain this criticism whilst maintaining the concept of "fixation point", another very useful Freudian notion to invoke in the psychopathological descriptions of our daily clinical practice, especially since this concept is conveniently linked to the fundamental problem of *regression.* In order to convince oneself of this, one only has to observe the considerable number of references to the concept of "fixation point" in psychoanalytic writings, according to the closely related *a priori* included in the concept of "stage". This, at least, is what I find troublesome in both cases, while recognizing the extreme difficulty in which one finds oneself when trying, in a clinical description, to do without this sort of anchor point, whose details can remain vague because it is assumed that everyone knows them, according to a consensus that remains implicit.

This is why I propose to develop here a different hypothesis, based on the constancy and the ubiquity of the instinctual drive pressure, which

Freud contrasts with the momentary and localized character of the external stimulus to which the subject reacts by muscular mobilization, by which he means the *striated* muscles. Thus, at birth, the libido cathects immediately, globally and in a diffuse way the psyche-soma of the subject-as-yet-to-come-into-being, with an immediately effective organizing valency of this cathexis *as much at the level of the genital organs as at the level of the digestive tract and its orifices – the mouth, anus and urinary meatus.*

The force of cathexis of the genital organs is due to the sexual quality of the libido, as well as to the cathexis, by those around him, of the child's sexual identity.

As for the power of the cathexis of the digestive tract and its orifices, it has its source in the immediate link that is established between the sucking reflex and the sensation – already internal – of hunger. A locus of early psychic cathexis, the digestive tract is from the outset a theatre of experiences that very quickly diversify. This is due both of the direct inaccessibility of its interior – governed by *smooth* muscles – and to the considerable difference, quantitative and qualitative, in the role that the stimuli provided by the external object play, depending on the orifices considered, which are governed, in their turn, by the *striated* muscles.

What are the advantages of such a model that is based on the physiological model and has already been utilized by Bion as a model in his psychoanalytic theory of thinking?

The first experience of the cathexis of the entire digestive tract may be considered as being located in the double register of the sexual impulses and the ego impulses. It sets up a crucial model of psychic life, namely, the *spatio-temporal vectorization of psychic experience destined to become preconscious.* It is this experience that will play an organizing role in the development of the specificity of the oral, anal and urethral erogenous orifice zones.

Since there is indeed a clear and immediate chronology between the experience of the first feed and that of the first stool, I do not think that it is necessary to artificially establish another, later one, based on the mastery of the striated muscles of the anal and urethral zones. This mastery can be considered as a later stage of an already organized/organizing instinctual drive cathexis.

On the other hand, I think that the orifice zones, whether oral, anal or urethral, can only be organized in a meaningful and differentiated way by means of a global and immediate libidinal cathexis of the internal space that connects them and *"forces" time and space into human beings* by means of this subjectively long and often painful intermediate stage constituted by the processes of digestion.

It is due to the sexual nature of the libido that the functioning of the digestive system has been able to take on such a complex valency of cathexes in humans. As it is a meeting place par excellence of ego drive impulses and drive impulses with a sexual aim, the development of unconscious representations concerning it and its orifices will have to undergo a considerable work of differentiating elaboration and will come up against many defences.

According to my hypothesis, it is on the basis of this global drive cathexis of the digestive tract organized by the temporality of the first digestion, that the following elements will be simultaneously differentiated, in addition to the *inside* and the *outside* of which Freud speaks:

1 The specificity of the oral area as a locus of the instinctual drive cathexis of the first relationships with an external object.
2 The specificity of the anal zone and, to a lesser degree, the urethral zone, as places for exercising control over the possession and expulsion of the internalized object.
3 The specificity of the digestive zone as a locus of multiple and mysterious subdivisions with regard to their drive cathexis, where the more or less elaborate exchanges of the subject with his internal objects take place in the very fabric of unconscious phantasies, in the issue of mourning and of the birth of thought.

Given that the functioning of the digestive system is indissolubly linked to the subject's physical survival, it is quite natural for it to serve as a model of functioning for the survival of his psychical apparatus.

Through its vital union with the oral orifice, the breast, which Freud referred to as the first object of cathexis outside the body, gives impetus to the subject's relations with the outside world by means of the basic mechanisms of projection and introjection and in accordance with the two principles of psychic functioning, pleasure/unpleasure and reality. The importance of the role of the maternal object has been extensively described by Winnicott (1960) with the concept of the "good enough mother" – which I like to translate as the acceptable mother – as well as by Bion (1967) with the concept of "mother's capacity for reverie". It is to be noted, however, that the latter specifically considers the impact on the infant psyche of the psychic qualities of the mother's adult Oedipal organization, qualities which, in Winnicott, remain interwoven with the material aspect of maternal care. Furthermore, throughout her work, Klein from 1921 to 1945 (Klein, 1975) richly developed the hypotheses with which we are familiar concerning the importance of the evolution of the relationship with this very first object of external cathexis with regard to the organization of the internal psychic world of the subject.

During the first digestive experiences, the *outside* will be confusedly experienced as a strange and inaccessible space, distinct from the *inside*, if only by virtue of the difference between maternal responses to the infant's distress. Indeed, though the best of mothers can offer direct satisfaction in the form of food to calm the needs, if not the desires, linked to orality, she will only be able to intervene indirectly and in a delayed manner over time when the infant suffers *inside* his digestive tract. The "cleansing" function of the mother only brings partial and external relief, and the infant will have to wait for what will seem a very long time for the effect of a possible relief from stomach aches that he may find hard to avoid experiencing. The disarray linked to the solitary experience of the *time of digestion* will participate in the *de-idealization* of an object that is both omnipotent and not distinct from the subject.

The mutual misunderstanding that thus develops is likely to generate a revival of defensive idealization to fight against the experience of breakdown (Winnicott, 1960), and at the same time constitutes a powerful engine for the infant's processes of projective identification towards the caring object, which is lost no sooner than it has been found.

Simultaneously with the organization of the cathexis of relations in the oral zone, dominated by introjective mechanisms, the anal zone, the cradle of auto-erotic cathexes, will develop, both under the impact of projective mechanisms and in a partially autonomous economy regarding the external object, while the urethral zone will as it were be annexed by the genital cathexes and the digestive tract will continue, as best as it can, its transforming function as an apparatus for "thinking thoughts" (Bion, 1962b).

It is usual to relate the most severe psychopathologies to early disorders of the cathexis of the oral orifice as an orifice directly dependent on an external object: merycism (Kreisler, Fain & Soule, 1966), anorexia (Kestemberg, Kestemberg & Decobert, 1972), very serious object relationship disorders, such as autism, psychosis and, to a lesser degree, addictive pathologies.

In contrast, the instinctual drive cathexis of the anal orifice is generally evoked in well-defined regressive configurations, essentially organized around the two main axes formed by perversion and obsessional mechanisms. In these configurations, dependence on the reality principle and on the external object is denied, while the object is taken hostage in order to serve defensive phantasies involving idealization of the subject's capacities and omnipotent control over the objects whose unacceptable mourning is dealt with by denial.

Contrary to these general theoretical views, our daily clinical practice reveals the inextricable complexity of pathologies of cathexis and the randomness of *fixation points*, even if reinforced by trauma, in our understanding of the analytical material and in our therapeutic objectives. The processes of *regression*, which are so polyvalent in any analytical treatment, seldom relate to a single point of fixation except in an ephemeral way, unless it is an optical illusion on our part, when we are faced with a condensation of phantasies that is too "dense" to be decipherable. In reality, pathology is always related to the *links* that are at the origin of meaning, much more than the *places* connected by these links. In support of this observation, I would point out that the attention paid, during an analysis, to confusional states, be they mild or severe, temporary or lasting, constitutes a therapeutic lever of choice to enable us to grasp the nature of the intrapsychic conflict.

It is within this perspective that I would like to situate the hypothesis of the *digestive model* that I am developing here, a model of linking between orifices that makes it possible to organize their specificity according to an immediate chronology. It is my contention, then, that the superficial observation that gave rise to the theoretical construction of an "anal stage" of relatively late onset was, in reality, induced by an error of perspective, and that it is the extension of this same error which, for the sake of consistency, isolated a so-called "oral stage" prior to the previous one. Indeed, if we start from the assumption of an immediate instinctual drive cathexis of the entire digestive tract, the apparent autonomy of a cathexis of both the oral and anal zones is, in reality, a deferred effect.

Long before the young child manages to control his sphincter muscles, subject/object differentiation and the cathexis of the Oedipal third element will already have been established. In addition to my experiences of infant observation and the numerous studies published in the field of perinatality, I need only mention the suddenly furious look of my son and, two years later, the suddenly fascinated look of my daughter when, one evening like all the others, a little after the end of feeding and the ordinary ritual of "burping", I passed them from my arms to those of their father who came, as usual, to join us after work. Both were about three months old. Though there may have been "stranger anxiety" in the sense of René Spitz (1965), this "stranger", so well accepted until then as an extension of the maternal object, suddenly and irreversibly took on the significance of the Oedipal rival for the boy, and of the Oedipal object of desire for the girl. The indisputable participation of the Oedipal organization of each of the two parents does not, however, account for the suddenness of the reorganization of the object cathexes in each of the two children. Now this reorganization, which may be considered as a key moment in the development of nascent thought, took place in direct relation to *digestive functioning*, set in motion by feeding. We cannot therefore validly rule out the role of the instinctual drive cathexis of this digestive functioning in the constitution of an analogical model having led, in the examples considered, to the sudden new significance of the Oedipal object.

Thought processes, an instrument of active control extremely rich in instinctual drive activity, which are organized along the lines of digestive processes, therefore act very early on as an antagonist to the "passive pleasure" invoked by Freud with regard to the first anal stage. Moreover, he equated this passive pleasure with female pleasure, with the intention of offering an interpretation of femininity that reduces the latter to the schema of male infantile sexual theories. The hypothesis of such an early and global cathexis of the digestive tract is quite naturally congruent with the concept of *après-coup* and all that it implies in terms of permanent conflictuality between the sexual drive impulses and the ego-drive impulses.

This is why I think that the child's interest in his faeces, which can be observed when he reaches the age corresponding to the description of what is called the "first anal stage", constitutes one of the auto-erotic vicissitudes of his processes of thought and symbolization, involving an oscillation between its positive and negative aspects. It is perhaps during this period of human life that we can get the best measure of the psychic prematurity of the human infant and identify the independence of the instinctual drive equipment and its organizing force, in contrast with the state of physiological dependence.

By the time the child is actively interested in establishing adequate sphincter control, characteristic of the "second anal stage", the instinctual drive cathexis of his thought processes and his capacities to express them by means of adequate symbolization will have already grown considerably. As Alain Gibeault (1989) has shown, the number and diversity of observations concerning the implementation of these processes show, on the one hand, that they appear very early on, and on the other that they concern spoken language immediately, simultaneously with images. It is precisely this psychic complexity that allows the young child to give up passive dependence on maternal cleansing care, and to start experiencing with sufficient pleasure the reality of a new autonomy – the closure of his body space – thus acquiring a certain mastery over his feelings of repletion and intensifying his projective identification with the maternal alternation of gifts and frustrations. So the seemingly dominant interest that the toddler displays for his sphincter control is therefore only one of the manifestations of his instinctual drive cathexis of mastery (Denis, 2002) over both external reality and thought, along with its verbalization, as well as his voluntary motor skills.

The infant Oedipal organization of the fourth year of life, as discovered by Freud, is another key moment in the reorganization of instinctual drive cathexes under the influence of the fascination that perception of the reality of the adult couple, whether homosexual or heterosexual, who are raising them, has on children; this perception has now become unavoidable and takes them back, without any possibility of escape, to their original phantasy of the primal scene. At this age of constantly asking "why?", the child tirelessly defends himself against the only question to which he intuitively knows, in the upheaval of the Oedipal catastrophe, that there is no answer: how does the love that these adults give each other differ in quality, libidinally and emotionally, from that which he gives and receives from them?

Underpinned by the predominance of the genital aspects of drive derivatives in thought activity, the language-based symbolization of which is now firmly acquired, the renewed sexual excitement expressed by children of this age comes from the asymptotic gap that henceforth exists, throughout their lifetime, between that question and its lack of an answer. It is only at this price that the "why" of the primal scene remains the ferment of all evolution and discovery. But, as he will do later through more or less sublimated activities, the 3- or 4-year-old child invents all kinds of false solutions in order to seek the unattainable part of the truth but also to hide the part that he understood right away and that tears him apart: they love each other and, in their exchanges, something ineffable and unrepresentable happens that the child can neither give nor receive.

For the subject that concerns us here, I will argue that both the hypercathexis of the non-genital orifices albeit designated as erogenous zones, and the construction of infantile sexual theories with phantasies of exchanges, between the parents, of good or bad food, a good or a bad penis, good babies or "pooh-babies", fall for me into the category of what Robert Barande (1989) called "lies to oneself", lies from which we hope to derive consolation without really believing in it much – at least in the case of normal libido development. This is where the anchor point of the castration complex lies, in the diachrony that governs its components, in boys and girls respectively.

Through the essential reorganization of this Oedipal period, the libidinal cathexis of the digestive tract and its orifices meets the limits of its conceptual formalization in the impossible and forbidden aspects of adult love. The ego-impulses will reinforce the cathexis of the image of the adequate and autonomous functioning of a castrated – that is to say, asexual – body, while the sexual impulses, to which auto-erotic satisfaction will suffice less than ever, will be forced increasingly to follow sublimatory and identificatory paths. Under the simultaneous and contradictory pressures of the *renunciation* of Oedipal wishes – linked to the principle of reality definitively establishing the difference of generations – and of the *repression* of these same unfulfilled wishes, these various cathexes will find expression in a multitude of new forms, organized in a more visible way in defences against the primal scene.

The material of Little Hans (Freud, 1909) gives us some illustrations of the complexity of representability in connection with the development of his phobia. Thus, the horse's head, with its blinkers and the piece of black leather on its muzzle, may be understood as a phobogenic object insofar as it represents both a paternal image and a "combined object", a faecalized reducer of the primal scene. Likewise, the little boy's passionate interest in his mother's urine and faeces forms a contrasting pair with his disgust for her yellow and black drawers. Hans' curiosity about the difference between the sexes makes use here of the displacement permitted by both his external entourage and his internalized superego. This displacement continues in the image that he communicates to his father, when he tells him that he wanted to "do lumf" when he saw those drawers.

It would have been far more dangerous for Hans to have spoken of an erection, or even to experience an erection in this instance. The repression therefore protects the little boy's sexuality, while the return of the repressed manifests itself in the "asexual" sphere of the digestive configuration. Hans was to be prohibited from having an erection again when he was forbidden from climbing over the boxes on the luggage-cart to reach the loading dock of the warehouse. Hans' confidence in the reliability of the support of the paternal penis in this exploration of the maternal sexual organs is understandably corroded by the mixture of exciting/excited inquisition, lies and interpretive violence that the latter forces him to undergo. Under these conditions, his Oedipal rivalry and his castration anxieties, undoubtedly present, are difficult to observe in their natural state. His fear of being carried away by the cart without being able to get off it in time may, however, be interpreted as his fear of the intensity of his genital impulses. He quickly reassures himself by means of regression: "I can always come back to Mummy, in the cart or in a cab". But he adds, "I don't know [what I'm afraid of]), but the Professor'll know. *D'you think he'll know?*" (Freud, 1909, p. 48; my *italics*]. Hans begins to get used to the idea that adults refuse to accept that children are capable of possessing or acquiring knowledge, starting with the knowledge that the child already has and about which he would like to communicate. The de-idealization of parental imagos is painful and, here too, withdrawing to the level of digestive functioning helps to restore the parental coat of arms with a little idealization.

It remains for me to examine the fate of the link that exists between the unconscious fundamental phantasy of the primal scene and the Oedipal return of the repressed; this last secondarily sexualizes this digestive configuration at the end of the Oedipal period *within the framework of the state of mind characteristic of the latency period*. Indeed, this state of mind constitutes, not only in the child but also in the neurotic adult patient, a privileged regressive scene, a "stage" of choice on which to portray multiple scenarios, and where, on the theme of primitive scene and under the guise of the digestive model, infantile sexuality is reorganized retroactively.

The anal orifice thus constitutes, *for the little boy only*, the locus of displacement of the repressed vagina through which he imagines in phantasy that he is entering the maternal body, while *children of both sexes* can pretend that they came out of it as a locus of displacement of the uterus, an even more repressed aspect of female sexuality, which I have explored (Guignard, 1997b) in my study of the adolescence of femininity. The anus ensures the coherence of such an infantile sexual theory since it constitutes the way out of a digestive system whose mouth represents the path of entry to fertilization. This is another means for the infantile preconscious to kill two birds with one stone by reduplicating its repression of the vagina while maintaining the presence of an oral cathexis which it had inevitably been led to mourn as a result of weaning.

The digestive configuration conceived as an irreproachable defensive organization benefits from a considerable period of time before the post-pubertal reorganization to establish presuppositions whose advantage is that they have the coherence of an apparently innocent logic. Its aspect of devitalizing obsessive control is particularly active throughout the period of latency, while at puberty it once again becomes more clearly the preferred mode of expression of a stammering genital sexuality that is too exciting in its unknown sensory and relational perspectives to be easily integrated. We will find it at work in adults, both in obsessive and homosexual issues and in certain thought and behavioural disorders, where it manifests itself in alliance with group mentality, the components of which I have examined in other studies (Guignard, 1994b).

To take up the dissociation, proposed by Meltzer (1973) of the Freudian formula according to which "the young child is a polymorphously perverse", it is worth noting finally that the *digestive configuration* lends itself very well to the representation of both the *polymorphous* aspect and the *perverse* aspect of infantile sexuality. The famous tale by Grimm of *Hansel and Gretel* offers a metaphorical illustration which I will outline by way of conclusion.

> When they go out to collect wood with their poor parents who are at the end of their resources, Hansel and Gretel, two children, brother and sister, are intentionally lost in the forest by their parents. Helped by the animals of the forest and guided by numerous magic clues, they finally discover a clearing in the centre of which is a gingerbread house. Beginning to devour it with gusto, they are surprised by the witch who lives there. The witch coaxes them into entering her house where, once locked up, they face a very sad fate: the witch places Hansel in a cage and burdens Gretel with all the household chores, but in particular, she forces Hansel to eat so as to fatten him up for a delicious roast. Fortunately for the two children, the witch cannot see anything, and they are very clever: day after day, through the bars of his cage, Hansel holds out a chicken bone to the witch instead of his finger to show how his fattening is progressing. But the moment arrives when the impatient witch decides she cannot wait any longer to eat Hansel. The terrified Gretel is forced to prepare the fire in the stove, but she suddenly has a brilliant idea: as the witch asks her if the stove is ready, the little girl pretends not to know and, inviting the witch to come and take a closer look, pushes her into the stove where she disappears in the flames. Once free, the two children discover sumptuous treasures

> that once belonged to the witch, seize them and find their way home. Their father, who has since become a widower, now lives alone and is delighted to see his dear children again. All three lead good lives by shamelessly spending the witch's treasure.

Morality, in the form of an interpretive dream:

> The feeling of hunger is sometimes difficult to distinguish from sexual excitement, which drives us, "me-little-boy" and "me-little-girl" – that is to say "me-in-my bisexuality" – to go and see what is happening in the maternal forest. But these wicked parents keep their intimate life to themselves and leave us all alone, in the night of our desires; we are guided only by our animal instincts and a certain degree of magical thinking. So, we dream that we succeed in discovering the vaginal clearing, the gateway to all the treasures of the maternal body. But we do not have the means to enter it: it is only a dream, and we have *forgotten* – repressed – this ineffable intuition of what we cannot achieve. To console ourselves, we decide that this place must be like our behind, *which we know very well.* We imagine that we can acquire and share all these good things that parents keep for themselves, which must appease this burning sense of hunger-excitement. In particular, we do not want to admit that, despite the explanations that we have been given, we have neither the right nor the means to achieve it, so we imagine that it must be like this gingerbread, *which we know very well,* because we receive it, once a year, at Christmas. Me-little-boy is very glad that Daddy is not there and so will be able to "eat" Mummy all by himself or, if need be, give a little to me-little-girl if she is nice – well, something that we decide is like "eating", *which we know very well,* because, to be honest, what we have an intuition of is beyond our reach. Besides, the dream goes wrong since, even when sleeping, we know that we are too small, incapable of and forbidden from enjoying these adult pleasures. Mummy, who seems to be kind during the day, forbids us, in fact, from participating in the sexual feast as well as from staying alone together in order to excite each other i.e. by myself. As for Daddy, he has made himself inaccessible: so he must agree with Mummy. Me-little-girl is desperate because Daddy has disappeared. It is surely this witch/mother who has "eaten" him and, moreover, now she wants to keep me-little-boy for her personal use. It's me-little-girl who has to play Cinderella – please forgive the reference! – while she, the witch, is tending to his every need. But me-little boy is beginning to be afraid: me-little-girl tells him that the witch prefers him and so will surely "eat" him, just as she must've eaten Daddy – or his penis – and me-little-boy therefore has an interest in posing as a "little-chicken" – regression – to

avoid such a disaster – castration. Fortunately, there is me-little-girl, who seems less dangerous to me-little-boy than this mother/witch, and who seems to loathe her intensely. As we have already got rid of Daddy, let's also get rid of Mummy, and like that we will have all the treasures that Daddy gave her for ourselves, all those babies/jewels that she must've hidden in her "coffer/behind". . . . Finally, it is me-little-girl who has the last word in the dream, since we find Daddy again. But me-little-boy is so much stronger and richer than this poor castrated Daddy! So it will be us, the children, who will triumph over these poor pathetic parents and their old-fashioned genitality!

Note

* A first version of this chapter was published in the *Revue française de psychanalyse*, 1995, 59, 3, pp. 771–784 (Guignard, 1995b).

Chapter 13

Sexual life and identificatory reorganizations in adolescence

The Oedipus complex in adolescence

The adolescent version of the Oedipus complex is classically considered to be the result of a profound reorganization of the relations between the three agencies, that is, the id, the ego and the superego – which, according to the second theory of the Freudian topography are constitutive of the psychical apparatus of a subject – and their relations with external reality. This reorganization implies *de facto* a new series of modifications in the unconscious relations of the ego of the adolescent[1] subject with his internal objects and, first and foremost, with those that constitute his superego. It is also worth pointing out, from the angle of the first Freudian topography, that the *Pcs.* of the adolescent subject is forced, due to the pressures of biological growth on the one hand and of the *socius* on the other, to carry out a considerable reorganization of its relations with the *Ucs.* and the *Cs.*

This *Pcs.*, a psychic skin whose osmotic function regulates the exchanges between psychic life and external reality, will normally become, for a while, more "transparent" and more fragile, while the subject will modify more or less radically his attitude towards the world.

Adolescence, a luxury (sub-) product

Many psychoanalysts (M. & E. Laufer, 1989; Cahn, 1991; Alleon, Morvan & Lebovici, 1990; Baranes, 1993; Ladame & Jeammet, 1986) have emphasized the importance of the modifications that take place in the subject during the processes involved in forming his ideal objects, in the second part of adolescence, and in particular with the onset of a more or less regular sexual life. For my part, I have suggested that the full development of the period of adolescence and the adolescent mentality be considered as the product of the socio-economic and cultural luxury of the rich – so-called developed – countries (Guignard, 1988) I subsequently put forward the idea that one of the essential parameters of every form of human social organization consists of problems related to the management – and even the avoidance – of the huge work of mourning of the relationship with the first libidinally cathected objects (Guignard, 1989).

By way of extending these reflections here, I would like to add that the apparent erasure of the characteristics of the period of latency in favour of an illusory advance of psychic puberty over biological puberty may be considered as a phenomenon revealing the decadent phase of every civilization that has previously attained the stage of writing. This phenomenon – which thus concerns both sociology and psychology – modifies, in my opinion, the generally accepted classification which distinguished a first, and then a second period within adolescence.

Today it is fair to consider that adolescence as a characteristic process of the identificatory and symbolic reorganizations increasingly tends to be confined to what is generally called the second part of adolescence. Indeed, contrary to what occurs in other kinds of civilizations, where the break between childhood and adulthood is marked by rites of passage expressing its ineluctable and irreversible nature, the children of the three last generations in the West have lived, and continue to live, in a family and social reality that favours, if not provokes, the establishment of a long period with ill-defined boundaries.

This period covers, on the one hand, the period of "latency" in the Freudian sense of the term, even if it has not retained the basic characteristics of post-oedipal repression and, beyond the period of puberty, of the first period of adolescence.

The period during which the human infant is thus, if not protected, at least essentially incapable of taking care of himself, also constitutes a prolongation of the period of ambiguity in his sexual identifications, which has primordial consequences for the status of the individual as the subject of his own existence.

This prolongation contains two possibilities of avoidance, one concerning the recognition of the difference between the generations, and the other, that of the difference between the sexes. The pleasure, or even the narcissistic complacency with which the preceding generation contemplates the way adolescents disregard their situation in the generational line and their sexual affiliation will enable them to avoid as far as is possible the painful *work of solitude* that awaits every evolving subject. Thus, the longer the period of time that is given by a society to the young individuals who belong to it to try to negotiate the mourning of their primordial objects, the more this negotiation risks veering towards avoidance. At the same time, the nature and qualities of the identifications that result from it will be modified according to parameters of which we currently have a very limited view.

Even if the period of latency no longer has the rigidly structured aspects that it once had, it remains – and will do for some time yet – the privileged moment during which the forever moving relationship between the projective and introjective registers can be restructured and stabilized. And if puberty no longer consists necessarily in this solitary discovery of a newly acquired sexual body, it remains nonetheless the period of the uncertain encounter with a future rendered present in the reflection of the mirror.

It is at the level of the first period of adolescence that social changes make themselves felt most clearly: indeed, this period no longer corresponds to the days when pubertal children, aged thirteen or fourteen, left family and school to learn a trade and work as adults. This period in which family and social models were integrated or rejected with a rapid and sometimes limited flowering of the capacities of symbolization, has lost its specificity with the prolongation of the obligatory period of schooling, thus complexification on the one hand and de-differentiation on the other, which today burden the working world with a degree of inactivity that is troubling. This first period of adolescence has thus become, more than ever, the privileged period of the false-self and of pretence for the young adolescent who utilizes his status as a part-object, an object of commerce or a fetish – thus a sub-product – to maintain what are often very violent relations with a society which exploits above all his infantile omnipotence.

This is why anyone who still has the project of rediscovering the authentic nature and specific psychic organization of adolescence currently finds himself reduced to focusing more specifically on the terrain of the second period of adolescence. It is there only that one can hope to study in any detailed way the reorganization of the cathexes and identifications of adolescent subjects.

Yet we are also confronted here with a particular scenario in which these older adolescents often live in more or less stable partnerships, even in their parents' home, with no legal or financial obligations imposed on them by the latter. This new state of affairs in no way presents the solid structuring of "enlarged families" living under the same roof, as often existed in the past, which have gradually disappeared, even in rural areas. In fact, the organization of which I am speaking here is one of the "provisional arrangement that persists", since these young couples live in a situation of random and temporary sexual promiscuity under the roof of the parental couple – or of the single parent – even when no material obligations oblige them to do so; and there again, it would be worth reflecting on the fact that there nearly always remains a margin of choice.

It is only when they come to think in turn about founding their own family, that is, in procreating, that an internal break between the childhood state and the adult state will perhaps take on its constrictive, and thus significant, character for these older adolescents. It is only then that they will have to give up their relative certainty as to the nature and qualities – positive or negative but, in any case, known – of the objects of their infantile pregenital and genital desires, and to tackle what I have called "the relation of uncertainty", the object of which will be that of the adult genital desire which has become accessible biologically, yet still remains for a long time psychically unknown.

Identification and symbolization at the end of adolescence

Whatever they have done with this suspended time that is the first period of adolescence, whatever they have done with their partnerships while still living with Mum and Dad, it is thus always the perspective of the following generation that constitutes the major occasion for a relational/identificatory reorganization in adolescents.

As it is essentially an unconscious process, *identification* has complex relations with *imitation* whose parodic aspect is chiefly observed in adolescence.

It is impossible, moreover, to tackle the question of identifications without taking into account its expressive means of support, namely, the *capacity to symbolize.*

Biological maturity plays a double role in adolescents, both disorganizing and reorganizing, disintegrating and reintegrating vis-à-vis the self-image, and it is at the level of the image of the adolescent's own body that the first experience of these modifications will be felt.

The body image

As the ego, according to Freud (1923a, p. 26), is "first and foremost a bodily ego", the battering inflicted by puberty on the previously established symbolic and imaginary organization will bring about a profound reorganization of the body image. Clinical experiences teaches us that, in adolescents, multiple symbolizations co-exist, which are true for some and false for others, of their transformed body (Schmid-Kitsikis, 1995).

We can observe three paths of expression and clarification of this question of bodily modification and its symbolized representation, each of which can range from the most normal to the most pathological, and all three can be used conjointly or not. These three paths are: *somatic expressions, psychic expressions and addictive expressions.* I have only distinguished them from each other for the sake of clarity of exposition, though in fact they overlap naturally.

Somatic expressions

Somatic expressions can be severe and fixed or benign and changing. They all have in common the fact that they aim to avoid, to distort, and even to expel all work of representing sexually the body of the subject who has become biologically adult.

Among the psychopathological configurations that can be classed in this category, we may mention: arrested physical development, anorexia, bulimia, dysmenorrhea, cystitis, severe skin allergies, but also sometimes extremely serious infectious illnesses indicating a sudden collapse of immune defences.

These diverse affections, whose degree of diagnostic and prognostic severity is highly variable, often set in following puberty. They are always accompanied by significant disorders of the body image, an image that may undergo such important splitting that, for instance, a pregnancy can reach its term without the "patient" or the medical team being aware for a single moment that she is pregnant, since they are so caught up in another body image because the patient is suffering from a serious illness with a severe risk of progression (Arnoux & Jean, 1985). In all cases where severe somatic expressions are encountered, we also observe an evacuation outside the mind of the representation of the image of oneself as a body that has become biologically adult.

In every case there is a split between a problem of identification of a "secondary" oedipal turn, on the one hand, and what I shall call a much more archaic and complicated "agglomerate", consisting of "bizarre objects" and "nonsense" (Bion, 1967). It is precisely this agglomerate that the analyst must examine in a very detailed way, striving to detect indications in it as to the nature and origin of what may have been expelled in this way from the mind and into the body by instinctual drive activity.

In my experience, we will inevitably discover a particularly active set of issues at the level of identifications with the objects-of-internal objects, some of which are "dead identifications".

Psychic expressions

Apart from the non-systematic somatic expressions of the post-pubertal conflict, more classically, psychic expressions can be observed, that is, a range of representations of the subject's body, representations that are sometimes highly symbolized and sometimes pseudo-symbolized, but which always concern a non-sexed and non-adult body.

Hysteria is obviously the typical example of this mode of representation, where the "innocent" infantile body makes its return instead of those aspects of infantile and adult sexuality that have been repressed, as Freud (1895) showed. Furthermore, in hysterical patients the return into the body is in the order of what has remained or has once again become regressively unsymbolizable for the subject, even though they reveal it all too evidently and in an illusorily meaningful way in their symptoms. It is one of the major difficulties in treating hysterical patients, for one may be tempted to interpret wildly a symptom that is so obvious for the observer, even though it remains totally foreign to them because it is split off.

Analytic interpretation should, on the contrary, make it possible to reduce this splitting and link up the broken threads of symbolization. There, too, it is important to determine the respective proportions of authentic expressions of the ego, on the one hand, and projective identifications on the other.

Quite different are the psychic expressions of the conflict in symbolizing the body that has become biologically adult in cases of *psychotic delusion*. It is the subject's entire identity that seems to have been smashed to pieces by the onset of puberty, because it is very often in puberty that severe forms of psychosis, in particular schizophrenia break out. There, too, the psychoanalyst finds himself faced with an "agglomerate" where there is "nonsense" (Bion, 1967). In my view, this nonsense originates to a large extent in the pathology of the internal objects which, having been projected outside, subsequently return in a delusional form.

Furthermore, while the *hypochondriac* adolescent maintains, by means of his constant complaining, an attempt to symbolize his conflict with damaged and persecuting internal objects, the adolescent suffering from a severe *intellectual inhibition*, which may signal the onset of schizophrenia, will cut off everything in his body image that risks forming a link with his objects, whether external or internal; I am thinking here, for instance, of catatonic states.

Addictive expressions

What can we say about addictive expressions of the modification of the post-pubertal body image? If I am regarding them as a distinct category, it is because, in my view, these expressions that I call addictive seem to me to be linked essentially to "group phenomena", a favoured mode of expression in adolescence, as we all know. I am referring to violence, drugs, dangerous sexual promiscuity and the ideologies which adolescents are fond of because they seek to diminish and even to suppress the differences that become increasingly unavoidable for them, at the level both of their own bodies and of the generations.

Now these addictive expressions as group phenomena constitute the ambiguous mode of defence against, and elaboration of, the symbolization of the adult body of the subject. Indeed, the group can serve as a mirror, either one-way or not, for the adolescent's newly acquired adult body.

Likewise, the group serves as a pseudo psychic skin for each of its members who mix and intermingle in it in a state of polymorphism flirting more or less with perversion, in the mad hope of avoiding for a little while longer the crucial challenge of individuation which identifies each one of us the inexorable solitude of human sexed (*sexué*) uniqueness.

What I am referring to here is not a pathological solitude – melancholic, for example, – but rather the unavoidable aspect of solitude inherent to all discovery, for every human being, of his own limits which make him a subject, an individual who is both alone and unique in his human condition, alone in entering into communication with others, alone in taking possession of his own thinking, through the reorganization, precisely, of the processes of symbolization in adolescence.

The relational/identificatory organization

Object-relating and identification are the two sides of one and the same process, which could be called "relational/identificatory", inasmuch as the relationship with external objects inevitably entails all or part of their internalization, in the most diverse states, within the psychic life of the individual.

Conceptualized in terms of part-object relations, the relations that exist between the different parts of the subject and the different parts of his objects of cathexis, both external and internal, are represented and symbolized in all their richness and complexity. It goes without saying that this work of representation must be carried out by every psychoanalyst who hopes to approach, symbolize and put into words for his patient the various identificatory movements, projective and introjective, between the patient and his objects.

The projective version of identifications implies a temporary abandonment of a part of the subject to the object with whom he identifies. The subject's sense of coherence is weakened, while he both enriches and encumbers himself with the "agglomerate" of characteristics of his object of identification. The novella by Julien Green (1949) *If I were you*, gives an admirable description of the increasingly vertiginous oscillations of the sense of self implied by a process of projective identification pushed to its extreme limits. In her psychoanalytic study of this text, Klein (1957) clearly showed the impoverishment of the subject's ego caught up in such a process of pathological projective identification. At the other extreme, we find the mother's capacity for reverie, which Bion (1967) made the prototype of normal projective identification.

As for *the introjective version of identifications*, I have already pointed out above that, like culture, it is what remains in the ego in the form of unconscious traces of a relationship with an object whose origin has been completely forgotten. Introjective identifications have their origin, I believe, in the early stages of individuation and of the early Oedipus complex, in particular during the "primary feminine phase" (Klein, 1932) of the fourth month of the first year of life. They accompany in a particularly intense way all the important moments of the reorganization of psychic life, in particular the Oedipus complex between the ages of three and four, puberty, the end of adolescence with the onset of adult sexual life, maternity for women, parenthood, then the mid-life crisis for both sexes and, more generally, all the moments of crisis and trauma requiring resolution.

However, in my view, they can only be formed in relation with projective identifications of good quality, while they will never be observed in organizations where pathological projective identifications predominate. These introjective identifications will form, and then enrich the very nucleus of the ego, based on the relations between this ego and its objects, both external and internalized. The introjective identificatory relationship may be considered as stripped of the essential elements of intrapsychic conflicts, while the ego leaves its objects to their own fate without interfering projectively.

In an earlier study, (Guignard, 1988), I suggested that the period of latency furnished the analyst with an excellent opportunity to help a subject consolidate the quality of his projective identifications and to favour a better equilibrium between the projective and introjective identifications. Considered from this angle and from the perspective of the pubertal reorganization of identifications with oedipal objects, child analyses in the so-called latency period seem to me to have an important prophylactic impact.

My position can be summed up by two central hypotheses:

1 Every normally constituted human being functions, from the age of around four to five months, simultaneously in the registers of projective identification and introjective identification, and does this throughout life. That is why every relational experience between a subject and an object of cathexis is likely to give rise to a *double relational/identificatory registration, one projective, the other introjective,* each of which is nourished by the relationship with the other.
2 The processes of symbolization have their origin and develop in this "double helix" of the communication between these two identificatory registers, projective and introjective. Thus the projective registration constantly takes hold of new aspects of the object and includes them in the relationship, while the introjective registration takes the passion out of, and gives greater flexibility to, the encysted conflicts.

It is this link between the two relational/identificatory modes with this or that object of cathexis, this *second-degree link* between the projective mode and the introjective mode of relating to the object, which, in my opinion, nourishes the subject's activity of symbolization through the connections between them of a multiplicity of representations of diverse origins.

This link, which is valid for all ages of life after individuation and the recognition of the otherness of the object at the level of the depressive position, will be enriched considerably in the aftermath of puberty, at the level of the number and categories of representations capable of being organized symbolically among themselves. These representations will in particular concern sexuality that has now become realizable and constitutes a danger that is not easily circumvented. The danger in question is of having to undertake without further delay the mourning of the parents of childhood, failing which development as a whole will be inhibited or arrested. For although key moments exist in this evolution of the processes of symbolization, the onset of adult sexual life probable constitutes the potential corner stone of it.

The relation of uncertainty and the regressive temptation

The perspective of acquiring this dangerous privilege linked to the adult genital capacity, a privilege that I call the "relationship of uncertainty" and that I regard as the specific feature of the relationship of the adult couple, constitutes a menace for the biologically mature adolescent at the level of his somato-psychic integrity.

Faced with this menace, the adolescent will experience particularly intensely the regressive temptation of infantile sexuality. In a movement of "reversal of perspective" (Bion, 1967), the adolescent will put his newly acquired adult capacities in the service of this regression, attacking more or less violently and in an organized way, with more or less perverse aims, everything that symbolizes his human condition, his affiliation to a determined generation and gender, thereby questioning the specific image of his sexual body and the reality of his human uniqueness.

Dress styles, make-up, hairstyles caricaturing the genital zones, tattooing, piercing, homo-or heterosexual overdetermination of jewels, ornaments, decorations, fetish objects, and so on, are all pseudo-symbolizations, false-objects imitating, derisively or murderously, the genital sexual relationship that has finally become accessible and, therefore, terrifying.

From this point of view, the group, the band, the gang and flaunted homo- or heterosexual promiscuity are all group formations whose mentality aims to caricature a plurality of cathexes, precisely when there is a lack of genuine multiple cathexes. This group mentality favours the fragmentation of cathexes, maintaining, moreover, by means of a confusion of genders, the illusion of a sexuality from which the projection in phantasy of a future generation is amputated. There is justification for speaking here of a cathexis of the penis as a phallic object – and not genital – which leads it very quickly, along the regressive path, to become a faecal penis.

The economic role of acting out and somatizations

All forms of identificatory and relational evolution run the risk of attendant repeated acting out, or even somatization. Two questions arise in this connection: how can this possible acting out and somatization be considered in terms of the quality of the subject's relational/identificatory links to objects, external and internal? Does this acting out and somatization present a specific configuration in adolescence?

The relational/identificatory links to objects

From the psychopathological point of view, it may be considered that acting out and somatization constitute fixation points determining the form and limiting the scope of regressive movements. That is to say, they also constitute "safeguards" (*garde-fous*), in the true sense of the word. From the point of view of the relational/identificatory links to the object, this acting out and somatization constitute proto-forms of cathexis which I call a "subject/object agglomerate". These proto-forms of cathexis occur essentially in the mode of projective identification which, when it functions too repeatedly and in an overly predominant way, can only become intrusive, or even pathological, ensuring for a long time that a genuine mourning of the object, and thus access to symbolization, is neglected.

However, this point of view is solely descriptive, and does not do justice to the elaborative possibilities contained in certain forms of repetition (Freud, 1914). Furthermore, this descriptive point of view characterizes neither the nature nor the qualities of the objects that are likely to be caught up in this subject/object agglomerate. In fact, these agglomerates are never of an oedipal/secondarized nature; rather they are comprised of old and vulnerable parts of the infantile self and of very archaic part-objects, bizarre objects, non-objects, objects-of-the object, dead objects, and so on.

In addition, the persistence of the acting out and somatization attending a mode of functioning in which projective identification of poor quality predominates can only be understood from the perspective of the existence of a pathological relationship between the object of cathexis and the internal-objects-of this-object, a relationship that it is the analyst's task to discover. Thus, the patient who is made attentive to the problem of the object-of-the object might formulate things as follows: "I suffer from the link that exists between certain aspects of my internal mother and of her own mother – or of her own father – within her". It is not a question of establishing a naively paranoiac "Babushka system", where responsibility is always rejected on to the previous generation in external reality. Rather, at the level of the theory of analytic technique, it is a matter of trying to understand, through the detour of the transference, and to describe to the patient the relational/identificatory links that exist between the analysand's internal objects and their own internal objects.

Experience shows that the patient emerges more quickly and more easily from states of confusion or unconscious pathological guilt when the analyst helps him to identify the psychic organization of the internal objects with which he is unconsciously identified, taking upon himself conflicts that are in fact those of the patient's internal parents with their own oedipal objects.

This particular technique of intervention favours differentiation between the pleasure principle and the reality principle; it helps the patient overcome pathological guilt and to acquire a sense of his real responsibilities towards himself and towards others.

Specificity and multiplicity of acting out and somatization in adolescence

Faced with the often-unforeseeable violence of the appearance of this symptomatology, and in the hope of being able to contribute in some way to finding better preventive measures, it is important to try to understand this mode of unconscious functioning of the adolescent, which seems to lead him, more often than not, to the edge of catastrophe.

Accession to biological sexual maturity reactivates and mobilizes anew the entire range of the adolescent's relations to his internal parents, in all the psychopathological complexity not only of the subject, but also of his internal objects. Acting out and somatization in the adolescent are indicative of a disorganizing regression of the capacity to symbolize under the impact of accession to biological maturity. Conflicts are telescoped within the adolescent's psychic life, and guilt may become so crushing that it must at any price be projected, either in the form of acting out, or into the subject's own body through somatization.

Thus, many resistances to treatment in adolescents are linked, in my view, to failures at the level of their internal objects, and especially at the level of their limited or inexistent capacities to see how a true relationship of affective intimacy is to be distinguished from acting out.

Accession to genital sexual life brings with it profound identificatory and relational modifications. The consequences of these modifications are felt at various levels and can be examined from the angle of the links that exist between the two relational/identificatory modes, the projective mode and the introjective mode.

Since the processes of symbolization are linked to this double registration, it is desirable to observe them very closely because they tend to deteriorate during this period of development, resulting in a resurgence of very strong unconscious guilt whose pathological aspects risk becoming interwoven with tendencies towards acting out and somatization. When an adolescent patient presents a significant tendency towards confusion, taking into account, in his analysis, the relations of his internal objects among themselves – "objects-of-the object" – makes it possible to relieve his extreme sense of guilt and, thereby, to favour the resumption of his processes of symbolization and identificatory relationships.

Note

1 The term "adolescent" is utilized here generically and includes adolescents of both sexes.

Chapter 14

The price of transformations in puberty

Who pays what?

Over the course of the 20th century and the worldwide conflicts that occurred during it, all societies underwent profound changes. Our western society was no exception. Its patriarchal base collapsed and methods of educating and teaching children underwent several revolutions. Around the world, the endemic rise of new technologies changed the way we look at the future and transmit our stories and cultures. In a slower and more discreet way, the human body also changed, as well as its relations with mental life which experienced, and still is experiencing, exciting and often trying discoveries.

As we enter the third decade of the 21st century, we must ask ourselves what the consequences of these changes are and how we can assess the lines of force that unite and differentiate both the soma and the psyche in today's children and adolescents.

Body and psyche

From the time of intrauterine life, sensory experiences leave memory traces in a memory originating in specific centres – notably the amygdala and certain temporo-parietal areas on the right side of the brain – which develop earlier than the centres linked to verbal memory, especially the hypothalamus. This memory is called "implicit memory". It concerns sensoriality and emotions, and will never spontaneously reach the status of the "explicit memory" studied by Freud, which is subject to repression. Mauro Mancia (2007), the Italian psychoanalyst and neuroscientist who died prematurely, proposed that we should consider implicit memory as the place where the unrepressed unconscious, as Jean Laplanche (1981) speaks of it, is stored. The sensory and emotional contents of this implicit memory underlie life during all developments of thought and action, all object relationships and all the identifications of the individual. They are part of the epigenetic equipment, bear the weight of the transgenerational, and also resonate with the "group mentality" (Bion, 1961) of the subject. Their importance surpasses the attempts made by verbal skills to put them into words. Like Freud, I consider that poets and artists are much more competent than psychoanalysts at creating an expression of it that accounts for the beauty and violence of life (Meltzer & Williams, 1988).

Whether we live briefly or for a very long time, our body and our psyche are condemned to live together until our last breath, and I think we are not always aware of the instinctual drive energy that this forced marriage requires at all times. We also do not measure the dynamics of the mutual sacrifices that they make to each other to maintain the coherence of a subject's identity that crosses so many different worlds, from its conception to its death. Finally, our science is still in its infancy in terms of listening to and interpreting the signs of dysfunction of this body/psyche totality. Due to his mammalian condition, the human infant remains in close contact with the maternal body for the nine months required – in principle – for its viability. At least, that is so when all goes well. Otherwise, the saving gestures are addressed to the body before anything else. Perhaps, only psychoanalysts will be able to hear, much later, after painstaking work and if they have listened very attentively, the effects on the psyche-soma, for example, of the noise of the machines whose action was necessary to keep alive a premature baby placed in an "incubator" (*en couveuse*) – the term is evocative of birds (*une couveuse* = sitting hen) and already involves the loss of body heat from mammalian mothers.

Towards the end of the 20th century, therapeutic attention, liberated notably (at least in the West) from the weight of perinatal mortality, gradually focused on the conditions of the transition of the foetus out of its aqueous medium towards the air medium in which the new infant will develop until he becomes an adult and lives "... the rest of his life", as the poet Joaquin du Bellay[1] says. We have discovered, or rediscovered, gestures intended to make this transition easier, thus trying to take into account the psyche as well as the soma, even if the scope of our certainties is still very limited compared to that of our hypotheses and constructions.

Since the second generation of psychoanalysts – if we consider that Sándor Ferenczi is already part of this second generation as an analysand of Freud – and jointly with the progress of clinical and developmental psychology, the interaction of the infant with his primary environment has become the object of great attention by child psychoanalysts, but also by proponents of the behavioural sciences. The mother of the newborn infant was considered the *deus ex machina* of the somato-psychic development of the little human being. Drawing inspiration from Winnicott, we repeated over and over again that a baby on its own did not exist; we focused attention on his notion of the "good enough mother (Winnicott,1958), as well as on Bion's (1967) notion of the "mother's capacity for reverie". I hasten to point out that I am one of those who pay the greatest attention to these developments, because I firmly believe that an adult psyche is essential for the proper initiation of the infant's capacity to think and for a harmonization of the relations between his body and his psyche. Not without concern, I want to draw the attention of the reader to the fact that in a period of surrogate mothers, artificial uteruses and "circular Oedipus complexes" rather than triangular (Ehrensaft, 2014), we will soon have to look at the personality of the sperm and the ovum, which would constitute a completely new and unprecedented chapter of our discipline – or its disappearance!

Anyway, there is a long way to go, before we can reconcile the relations between the body and the psyche and their respective developments, while seeking to develop as harmonious an interaction as possible between them. This interaction is essentially organized on an unconscious and preconscious level, and it is in the order of intimacy.

Intimacy

In my opinion, *intimacy* is an immediate and dazzling experience, which transcends social differences of age and gender. Its onset is instantaneous, when two people suddenly share *the same level of familiarity with a given sensory and/or emotional experience.* Intimacy is a transitory and ephemeral phenomenon. It can happen more than once between two people – or never again; if it returns, each occurrence will require from the two protagonists as much *intrapsychic openness and interpersonal availability* as the previous time. The life context and habits may or may not favour and support intimacy, but they never constitute it, in any way. A newborn baby does not have its own field of intimacy; rather, he participates in that of his mother. The advent of intimacy is congruent with the experience of the infant's introjection of a psychic container. With the feeling of having introjected a good object, which allows him to begin to constitute his ego and to live an existence which is his own, he will acquire a field of intimacy during the progressive introjection of the capacity for reverie and its skills of intimacy. The mother's sensory and motor attitude plays an important part in the intra-verbal communication that allows the creation of a field of intimacy in infants.

On the threshold of the depressive position, the discovery of the Other-of-the-mother pushes the infant to intensify his introjection processes in order to keep inside him what he is losing of the mother – or having to share – in the outside world. It is by internalizing this field of intimacy that he then discovers the existence of this same mode of relationship between his ego and his internal objects. Because of the importance of the part played by the body in the constitution of the ego, all bodily experience will quickly participate in the field of internal intimacy.

The infant's experience of his own body is the first and most enigmatic of these situations of intimacy, on the borders of the ego and the object, not only external, but also internal. Observation of babies and young children has familiarized us with the most visible of these relational manifestations, and psychoanalysis has recognized their drive component by establishing the concept of "auto-eroticism" – a concept that poses more questions than it solves, by the way, but that's another story.

I consider that the experience of intimacy depends greatly on the *epistemic drive,* which is part of the *third generation of the drives* (Guignard, 2015) as defined by Bion (1967): ±L, ±H and ±K. More specifically, the experience of intimacy is aroused by the intensification of the role played by the *primordial phantasy of the primal scene,* an intensification that is concomitant with the discovery of the mother's other object of love as a whole object, namely, the father – the metapsychological third. In order for L and H to be involved, it is therefore necessary to add an impulse of investigation, both with regard to this third object and, above all, to the emotions that it arouses in a mother whom the infant thought he knew well and whose feminine aspects he is now discovering, which are so different from the maternal aspects that were familiar to him (Begoin-Guignard, 1987).

The epistemic drive ±K derives its satisfaction from new discoveries in the register of the ego's relations with its objects, external and internal. In return, its functioning brings a revival of vigour, both to internal psychic life and to interpersonal exchanges. The most precious of these discoveries is that of a possible intimacy, not only between oneself and the other, but also – and perhaps above all – between the different parts of oneself, as expressed by the popular expression: "feeling good about oneself" (*être bien dans sa peau*).

A healthy functioning of intimacy provokes in those around reactions of "group mentality". For example, when a third person witnesses an intimate relationship, their Oedipal phantasies may provoke in them either a movement of "attack/flight", or a movement of "pairing" and "dependence" in a state of adhesive identification with the intimacy of the couple – or of the subject with himself (Bion, 1961).

Extimacy

Because of its position in the generations of drive impulses, the epistemic drive for an intimate relationship functions at the limits between the Self and the outside world. This is why we can consider it as an agent of interpersonal relations, which pushes the internal objects and the parts of the Self to seek in the external world an object with which relations of intimacy can be established. However, as we have seen, the quality of intimacy is rare and fleeting. We can therefore quickly find ourselves in situations of falseness and artifice, from which all intimacy has disappeared, employing its disguises and modes of behaviour. We may need a word to describe this psychic state, whose defensive valence must not be ignored, which can deny a real search for intimacy, too eroticised to be bearable for the subject.

This word was invented in 1923 by a French writer, Albert Thibaudet: disputing the denomination of "Journal intime de la France", given by Barrès to his *Chronicle of the Great War*, he wrote: "Le journal de la France? tout ce qu'il y a de plus *extime*!"

In 1979, another writer, Jean Echenoz, made Byron, his hero, a character

> without any tangible ties, without any special anchorage. Neither dwelling on objects nor décors, he traversed space with sincere inattention. He had never been able to acquire the concept of domiciliation, to conform to the civic imperative of the private, intimate, adhesive living space. . . . Thus, in Paris, his office on Boulevard Haussmann and his apartment on rue Pétrarque, the rigorous poles of a binary daily life, were also familiar and foreign, intimate as well as *extime*, similar in this, for example, to an elevator cabin, a dentist's waiting room, or a tobacco terrace on the Voltaire quay.
>
> (Echenoz,1979, p. 19)

Jacques Lacan (1969) once tried to use the noun "extimacy" (*extimité*), in his research on Freud's (1919) text "The 'Uncanny'". To the best of my knowledge, he did not continue to use it in his work.

Serge Tisseron (2001) has studied the phenomenon of *Loft Story*, and in this connection takes up this term extimacy; but he gives it a different meaning and opposes it to "exhibitionism". His description covers, in my opinion, that of the implementation of the epistemic drive in the mutual projective identification which functions in any search for intimacy with a new object. For this author, intimacy and "extimacy" constitute the systole and the diastole of self-esteem and the construction of identity. As far as I am concerned, I find this neologism particularly eloquent in describing the movement that transcends the boundaries of the private sphere, where intimacy is exposed to the outside, to the public, to the unknown, to the anonymous.

Finally: puberty!

Against his will, biological puberty is the first movement of "extimacy" for the future adolescent. Waking up with a broken voice, seeing hair growing all over your body, having nocturnal emissions, or even seeing your breasts growing and experiencing your first period, is to face the anxiety of becoming a stranger to yourself.

It is commonly held that with puberty, sexual arousal increases, and that its bodily locations become more precise. Except that we have observed for almost thirty years now a progressive disappearance of the latency period in western society, which implies that sexual arousal has hardly marked a break between the Oedipal period of between the ages of 3 and 5 and puberty, and that repression operates in a much less massive way than in Freud's time. We can hypothesize that such a change in the stages of growth of a part of the human species is due to what Piaget (1950) defined as an "anticipatory adaptation", which helps the prepubescent child to become part of a current western society that is openly excited by the bodies of its children in full pubertal transformation, a "youthfulness" to which advertising, the world of leisure and the professional world bear witness.

Today, alongside the multiplicity of sporting activities, our society also offers its young adolescents many opportunities to join groups and activities that flatter their omnipotence and their infantile omniscience – in particular by means of the "web". These opportunities encourage, in the pubescent child, the temptation to abandon responsibility for his own body, precisely at a moment when the latter no longer responds to the representations or the use that the child had of it hitherto. As a result, the pubescent child tends to make his body, and the image he has of it, conform to theoretically adult society. But the latter sees above all a mirror of its own adolescence, with its sexual excitement and its vulnerability, and too often takes advantage of the fragility of these budding teenagers, to seduce them with money, drugs, sex and violence.

Identity coherence varies from one moment to the next among those we call "teenagers". With new configurations, new defence systems appear, which lead them either to hide in a "claustrum" (Meltzer, 1992) of inhibition and secrecy, or, on the contrary, to use provocative exhibitionism in the hope of encountering the new limits of their body and their psyche.

Because the limits of their space of intimacy have been considerably shaken up by the process of puberty, communication on the web offers teenagers a pseudo-intimacy, which is nothing less, in fact, than an extimacy of their bodies, their feelings and their thoughts. Rather than alternating with movements of intimacy – as described by Tisseron (2001) – this extimacy arises in place of the task of mourning their childhood body, as evidenced by many videos on social networks, where we see girls at the beginning of puberty showing off the breasts that they do not yet have, during a pathetic and ridiculous "striptease", and boys trying to show off a rather shy erection, in circumstances of sexual seduction which leave the spectator rather doubtful. Faced with such images, a psychoanalyst will feel a particular compassion and concern for these children who thus expose themselves to a world full of dangers, hoping in vain to find a interlocutor who can contain their excitement and their anxiety at no longer recognizing themselves.

Extimacy does not deeply nourish a sense of identity. It only offers a momentary balm at superficial levels of self-esteem. "Being popular" is a very poor sweetener to replace the caloric components necessary to build a new identity coherence. The psychic transformation necessary to integrate our bisexuality requires lengthy work. The same goes for finding a good dynamic balance between intimacy and extimacy.

"I is another" (Arthur Rimbaud, 17 years old)[2]

Only a brilliant teenager could find such a poetic formulation to express the identity tsunami that engulfs the life of any child at puberty.

Faced with the invasion of the instinctual drives, the lines of splitting move, repression melts like snow in the sun, especially at the level of sensoriality. Far from uniting their voices with the genital valence of the sexual drive which has become insistent, the oral, anal and urethral aspects compete with it, each playing their defensive partition, seeking to externalize, in new appearances and customs, a little of the uncanniness that the pubescent child can no longer contain in himself. For some, the body pays the most apparent price – from piercings and tattoos to anorexia and self-mutilation. For others, it is the psyche that no longer "responds" – sudden and massive school failures, OCD and other obsessive behaviours, depressive breakdown, even an onset of schizophrenia. For others, it is addiction: alcohol, drugs, but also group sexuality and violence.

My goal is not to review here the psychopathology of puberty (Gutton, 1991), but to try to understand a little better the paths of impossible mourning that this reflects, and to examine the approaches available to us, as psychoanalysts, when we are consulted about it.

For the pathology of puberty is indeed a pathology of mourning, and if a literary illustration were needed, it would suffice to remember the metamorphoses of Alice in Wonderland,[3] who having grown in one big breath and is distressed because she can no longer see her feet which are now so far away, wonders how she will be able to keep in touch with them and exclaims: "I'll give them a new pair of boots every Christmas, with a message: *Alice's Right Foot, Esq., Hearthrug, Near the Fender, (With Alice's Love.)*" (Carroll, 1869, p. 16).

At the onset of puberty, the child loses the intimacy he had acquired with his body, first enveloped by maternal care, then forged by his sensory and motor experiences which have followed one another during the twelve or thirteen years of his life until then. This loss is often denied by parents, who see only their own loss of intimacy with a child who was still snuggling on their knees a few weeks ago, and who now withdraws into his room in exasperation, dragging behind him his long arms and interminable legs. The parents' phantasy is clearly sexual and, apart from often pathological exceptions, this leaves little room for an atmosphere of relational continuity which would be provided for a child who was allegedly "as before". And it is very understandable, because the body of the child who is becoming pubescent takes centre stage in the affective and emotional scene, creating an inexorable rift between him and the adults around him, who, themselves, maintain with their own bodies a continuity that is already old, dating from well before the birth of this child. The repression of the pangs of their own puberty obviously does not help matters.

Considered from the angle of identifications, this situation resembles a blocking of all mutual identification. The child feels like an alien, and I think that the fashion for monstrous toys, human/ animal/robot hybrids is not unrelated to a certain depiction of the difficulty of integrating the pubertal sexual urge with a child's body which, until then, had worked like a superb piece of machinery.

For their part, adults no longer dare to touch the child as they did before, in games or hugs, as this pubescent child resonates so much with their own puberty. If they still exist in the child's entourage, it is the grandparents who are the most capable relays to keep the affectionate current going and constitute an adequate excitation barrier to the fascination of the whole family for this new edition of human sexuality.

The attraction to outdoor spaces and events, sustained by the experience of a completely new state of adult sexual arousal, will quickly enter into conflict, in the mind of the pubescent child, with the comforts of family habits, if not of real intimacy. The family has become a space for projecting a past that the child has to grieve, including that of his familiarity and ease with his own body. Whatever it is, the family structure is no longer in tune with his internal whirlwind. A new balance between intimacy and extimacy must be found.

The child psychoanalyst faced with the patient's pubescent body

All the components of identity are therefore deeply disturbed by the onset of puberty, and such a disturbance also affects the environment of the child who has become pubescent. This is why the psychoanalyst cannot trust what parents say when they come to see us about their teenager: they could just as easily be speaking of a much younger child, rather than of this strange person he or she has become so suddenly.

The question of confidentiality is one of the most common issues raised when we are called to see a pre-adolescent in consultation, then in analytical psychotherapy. This parameter takes on a very particular importance insofar as the body and its pubertal transformations are both a major element and an almost absolutely unspoken element of the situation. I believe that I have always made sure that my patients can count on my discretion and reliability. Nevertheless, I have sometimes had to use my authority to share with the patient's entourage a crucial, even vital, element of what they had confided in me, regardless of their age. I have also sometimes transgressed civil law, by not reporting to the authorities a confidence that would have ruined the fragile transference relationship which was the only possibility of changing the dramatic situation of the patient for the better. In these situations, it is important not to confuse confidentiality with intimacy: whatever practical solution we adopt – or, more often than not, which is imposed on us from the outside – as regards our relations with the parents and relatives of a young patient, our only concern as psychoanalysts is to seek to establish a real relationship with the him or her, so that moments of intimacy can appear between us. By their yardstick, the confidentiality of all information received from those around them loses its importance: the data of external reality will always wash up on the shores of a true relationship of psychic intimacy between two human beings. I consider that, when a patient depends totally or almost totally on his entourage, the "fear of betraying him" that we evoke so as not to establish – and sometimes even seek – a relationship with this entourage on which he depends, emanates from a resistance on our side. The developments of the concept of intimacy which have taken place recently in the psychoanalytic community tie in with the clear distinction made by Donald Meltzer (1973) almost fifty years ago between intimacy as the expression of an adult genital mode of drive functioning, and the secret, which expresses a pregenital, and to be more exact, anal mode of functioning. As with any other patient, intimacy arises in a session with a teenager when the analyst is able to share a sensation or a feeling experienced, consciously or not, by the patient. This supposes that we are right at the heart of the psychoanalytic relationship. We will then be able to understand and, possibly, express these privileged moments in words at a later date. However, this intimacy rarely comes in the form of an obvious movement of sharing; it most often takes disguised forms, when one does not encounter a denial of what is happening.

Admittedly, a pertinent interpretation constitutes a specific and very useful tool in our search for intimacy. But such a discovery is rare, and it requires real work on oneself to achieve real sharing of the point of suffering and infantile helplessness in our patient. It is our countertransference that we must listen to, in the hope of making contact with this suffering projected into us by the patient, of experiencing it, rather than defending ourselves against it, which is our spontaneous reaction. Indeed, it is not uncommon that it is us, the psychoanalysts, who avoid intimacy for fear of feeling too close to our patients – and therefore too much sexual excitation. However, it is up to us to help our patient to be unafraid of the intensity of intimacy, regardless of his age and gender.

Along with "actings" – in and out – and enactments, somatic disorders are the most common defences against intimacy. These defences are mobilized whenever this relationship of intimacy regresses and "de-symbolizes", in order to be experienced by one or the other of the members of the analytical couple as a crude expression of the sexual impulses. However, whenever it is a matter of the body and its transformations, the risk of eroticization – and therefore of de-symbolization – is significant. What was already delicate in the relationship with younger children (Guignard, 2002) unquestionably takes on the appearance of seduction with teenagers. Sex education, at school and at home, does not make things much easier, because the difficulty is above all linked to transference, with its permanent movements of projective identification which promote erotic flare-ups, especially when sexuality becomes a theme in the session. Classically, it was recommended to choose a therapist of the same sex for teenagers, with the somewhat naive aim of favouring identifications with an adult of the same sex at the moment when the identity undergoes major upheavals. In fact, I have often found myself in a different situation – that is, of treating boys in puberty – and it is my experience that the work was achieved by integrating our own psychic bisexuality, and promoting the expression of the epistemic drive K. Today, in our post-gender era and at a time of the diversification and generalization of methods of medically assisted procreation and marriage for all, we will have to draw even more on the skills of our psychic bisexuality if we want to find out how to continue *talking about sexuality* with our child and adolescent patients from a place that can only be ours, unless it loses all its truth.

Time and space at puberty

The excellent lecture given recently at SEPEA by Isée Bernateau (2017) of the French Psychoanalytical Association (APF) titled "Lieux, non-lieux et anti-lieux à l'adolescence" nourished my reflections on the situation of space-time prior to adolescence, at the precise point of the temporal change that is puberty. Drawing on Gus van Sant's films on adolescence – the tetralogy of death – Isée Bernateau turned her interest to the importance of spaces during adolescence, a period during which time is stretched, distorted and sometimes reduced to a point, potentially final, namely, the death of the adolescent and/or his entourage. This allowed me to envisage a new point of view on the temporo-spatial "catastrophic change" (Bion, 1965) constituted by puberty, with a future abruptly revealed – the loss of his childhood body and of the parents of his childhood, while facing up to adult sexuality and a prospect of parenthood – while the proximate space remains the same for a few more years, but becomes falsely reassuring because it contains a new edition of the Oedipal conflict which is dangerously close to the crossroads of Thebes. We could understand the departure of Oedipus from the Corinthian royal family – unaware that it is not his biological family, but rather his adopted family – as a metaphor for the movement which increasingly takes the teenager away from his hitherto familiar family space. The murder of childhood – tragically carried out in the Columbine massacre which inspired Gus van Sant in his 2003 film *Elephant* – stops time, and it was the genius of the filmmaker to have substituted an almost infinite, deserted space for it. Because this is indeed a representation of the internal psychic space stretched, turned into a desert and rendered without limits by this temporal change which is inexorably coming and completely unknown.

I then wondered if there might not be a therapeutic lever to explore when we are consulted at the time of puberty about someone who is still only a child, but who carries within him the whole future of the world. I imagined that we could enter with him into an *emotional reflection* – this is the most suitable term that I can find – in connection with this temporo-spatial upheaval whose grave and tragic tone is far removed from the manic seduction exerted by society on the adolescent who is becoming an adult. We could then take a more accurate measure of how he feels about it, thereby decreasing the sometimes infinite space that separates us from him, also reducing his phobia of thinking – and ours.

Notes

1 "Happy is he who, like Ulysses, had a great trip, / Or like he, one who conquered the fleece, / And then came back, full of experience and reason / Living with his parents for the rest of his life", Joaquin du Bellay, Sonnet XXI, stanza 1, *Les Regrets*, 1553–1557 (Bellay, 1558).

2 "I is another. If the brass wakes the trumpet, it's not its fault. That's obvious to me: I witness the unfolding of my own thought: I watch it, I hear it: I make a stroke with the bow: the symphony begins in the depths, or springs with a bound onto the stage". Letter from the Seer to Paul Demeny, May 15, 1871. (From: http://rimbaudanalysis.wordpress.com/letters/) (Rimbaud, 1871).

3 See Chapter 6.

Chapter 15

Child and adolescent psychoanalysis*

The future of a reality

Night watchmen, for the love of the living world

The discoverers of psychoanalysis considered this new discipline as a science as well as an art. This was how medicine was described at the time. But nowadays there are few people who know anything about psychoanalysis other than in the form of a station kiosk caricature. The description of "scientific", which had only been attributed to it with a great deal of reticence, was promptly withdrawn with the advent of neuroscience.

As for art . . . who is concerned about it in the realm of science, in a century when research is invested above all in marvellous machines which can see everything inside us, except what is essential, namely the human person?

By way of example, apart from verbal memory, a sensory, preverbal and even prenatal memory, located in the subcortical zones of the amygdala and of the hippocampus, has been discovered. But to make use of this fine discovery, psychoanalytic thinking (Mancia, 2007) is needed, otherwise we cannot measure the long-term effects of an event, possibly traumatic, that occurred during this period of life which lasts, it is well to recall, for more than two years. Neuroscience is then improperly called upon to impose on contemporary research in the human sciences a scientism repudiated by the discoveries of quantum mechanics and combatted by many philosophers of science.

Child and adolescent psychoanalysis have always had their detractors, including amongst the ranks of psychoanalysts who confine themselves to analytic practice with adult analysands: admittedly, it is interesting to identify pregenital sexual impulses when these are repressed in an adult neurotic, but sitting on the floor to play with children who are going to dirty your nice office and who, moreover, are likely to ask you if they can use the toilets and may well need your help, is quite another matter. Let us be serious: Freud (1909) discovered infantile sexuality and the Oedipus complex; but we are not babysitters and these stories of breast and pee-and-poo are only interesting when reading Little Hans!

And yet there are psychoanalysts who consider that psychoanalysis is one and indivisible, and who persist in treating children and adolescents in the same way as adults. A handful of stubborn and recalcitrant practitioners, of whom I am one, – whose place within the psychoanalytic societies to which they belong varies from country to country – who proclaim their passion for the processes of development, the formation of the function of symbolization, the existence of transference in the child and of the Infantile in the adult and, above all, the conviction that psychoanalysis is, as Freud always asserted, a therapy, a *psychotherapy*, which is healing as much for the child and adolescent as it is for the adult, on the condition that one acquires serious training in each of these specific practices.

But there is also the society in which we are living; a society whose structures are cracking everywhere under the impact of deep and often obscure pressures – drive impulses in all their forms, including their trivial expression in the group mentality – pressures that are scarcely controllable with our weakened and obsolete means.

Nowadays human relations have become "something one has to manage" – but go and explain that to an infant in distress. And if a mother approaches her relationship with her newborn infant as if she were managing a property company, we need not be surprised by the damage that will be observed subsequently. . . . And yet, it can be observed on a daily basis: it is necessary "to be centred on oneself", to take "one's place" – and it's just too bad if one neither knows who one is or what this place is. What is essential is to advance towards a concrete aim, while looking neither left nor right to avoid the risk of feeling destabilized by discovering human distress around oneself. We must "manage our emotions" just as we manage a bank account: by only drawing small quantities daily from the cash-point, we will not run the risk of having our heart stolen.

On the other hand, where sexuality is concerned, it is seen as good form to display it, and even to exhibit it in its most basic forms of expression. Sublimation has returned to the chemistry laboratories once and for all and, when it comes to tenderness, we content ourselves with the "Annual Day of Cuddles". In other words, intimacy has a bad press – the word is not in use on the social media.

Finally, ideals are no longer of interest to any one, that is, as soon as they lie outside the domain of measurable performance. We may ask ourselves if they are not taking diabolical revenge for this disenchantment by attracting so many adolescents into the trap of paranoid group beliefs that drive them to murder and suicide.

Are there no longer any dreams, then? Ah? . . . that is to say . . . for a long time now we have known everything about the localizations and rhythms of dream activity – thanks to a certain, very interesting, Michel Jouvet (1992), even if he is not the great Louis[1] – but we still do not know much about the function of dreaming, except that dreaming is good for one's health. . .

Here, quite obviously, psychoanalysts could make themselves useful for interpreting these dreams. Likewise for fantasies . . . but this implies taking into account so many parameters and, above all, establishing links with the Infantile, all of which takes up a lot of time. But today we are in a hurry. Everything must be done very quickly, today's aim being to beat yesterday's record. Don't ask me why or I might speak to you about a phobia of death. . .

The Bubble

Fortunately, we have the Bubble.

The Bubble (with a capital B) appeared in the 1940s, in particular with Alan Mathison Turing (Girard, 1995) and the first formalizations of a brilliant system with two elements: 1–0, which permits an exponential combinatory system. The Bubble is a neo-reality whose scale and power go well beyond anything we could have imagined. After the (official) abolition of slavery, it has provided man with instantaneous help in all domains. From the point of view of culture, it has sidelined museums throughout the world and reduced the very large François Mitterrand Library to the rank of a curiosity cabinet. From the point of view of human relations, in two clicks it provides you with hundreds of thousands of "friends". From the point of view of the imagination, it presents the most terrifying monsters and invites you to enter the most phantasmagoric worlds – but not to leave them again. From the point of view of information, it tells you everything about everything; but distinguishing between genuine news and fake news, that is another matter.

Furthermore, online trading is in the process of ruining luxury shops as well as supermarkets throughout the world. The Bubble also benefits from the management of prostitution and pornography, as well as from ideological crime. No domain of interest, no area of human activity escapes it. In two clicks, one obtains the best and the worst.

The handling of this machine offering immediate satisfaction is simple: it operates according to the method of "trial and error", well known to ethologists. It was Serge Tisseron (2012), a leading expert of the Bubble, who told me this (personal communication) and since then I have been able to observe and confirm this for myself.

The general euphoria aroused by the scale of the applications of this discovery of the binary system is a state of mind that no one can escape, neither you nor me, nor anyone else. Too many dreams of humanity have found their material realization by virtue of it, and it would be ungracious of us not to be in awe of it.

Nevertheless, in spite of its fabulous performances, commercial but also reparative, the process of imitation contains within itself its own limits: imitating is not creating. Even "creations" in 3D are, *stricto sensu*, imitation.

In the classification of levels of intelligence realized by Jean Piaget, this method is characteristic of the level of concrete intelligence. One could not put it more clearly. It is worth recalling that Piaget's classification of intelligence levels places hypothetico-deductive intelligence at the summit of intellectual intelligence, thus, obviously, above concrete intelligence. It is to this higher level that creativity also belongs.

In the universe of the Bubble, this hypothetico-deductive intelligence is put in the service of the system of trial and error of concrete intelligence. It advises its technicians with the aim of creating new software models capable of imitating the subtleties of the states of a human soul. But will it succeed in integrating with robotics the *negative capacity* dear to Keats (Forman, 1952), to Bion (1970), and to us all? I very much doubt it.

Temporality and reality

Be that as it may, the greatest success of the Bubble lies undeniably in the fact that it abolishes time.

The words "when I'm grown up" are a thing of the past: children are much more skilful now than grown-ups in handling computer technology, and the notion of "parental control" is a tall story.

The restrictions linked to the opening hours of shops, historical monuments or administrations are over! Two clicks and you are on the site you want. After that, everything depends on the skills of those who have created the software programs, and a call for tenders for improving those of administrations would not be superfluous. . .

Are the metaphysical anxieties linked to the passing of time and death also a thing of the past? Is the plea of Alphonse Lamartine (1817) a thing of the past?

> O time! suspend your flight! and you, blessed hours,
> Suspend your swift passage.
> Allow us to savour the fleeting delights,
> Of our most happy days!

For with the poet, as with everything that is *living*, we are not governed by the binary system 1–0. We have rediscovered our temporal dimension. We have emerged from the Bubble, from this "nickel-chrome" neo-reality where death is as virtual as life. Time has caught up with us and, with it, anxieties, regrets, love and hate, and also uncertainty, the primary virtue of all scientific curiosity.

Here we are, then, back again in reality, in temporality and its mysteries, in truth also, with all its lures and its subterfuges, and also in our passion for discovering some fragment of it, constantly putting to the test our convictions and our beliefs, those beliefs that are the salt of our psychic earth, inseparable from the nucleus of our ego, forged by our very first introjections.

And that is what I was coming to: we all know that reality does not follow the law of the virtual world, but rather that of the living world. But have we appreciated the first consequence of this affiliation? Are we really conscious that a given reality does not always last? It is born, lives and dies, just like us.

In our defence, it should be pointed out that a human life is often too short to experience all the dimensions of a given reality. A collective effort is required that crosses generations, languages, cultures and beliefs. And yet I have often noticed that we could do better if we were not blinded and deafened by the compulsion to repeat. We would undoubtedly avoid some major errors if we were able to listen "without memory or desire" to our ascendants *and* our descendants.

A newborn infant does not fall passively into a ready-made reality. Each newborn is the bearer of a new part of reality. And, like each newborn, this new part of reality can be welcomed, loved, contained, cherished and raised. It then has a chance to deploy its capacities of transformation during its lifetime. This lifetime of a part of reality is not identical with the lifetime of the individual that brings it into the world but, like the latter, it is inexorably limited in time.

Alternatively, this part of reality may be subject to foreclosure (*Verleugnung*) and rejection (*Verwerfung*). It may be hated, neglected, ignored and left to its own devices, like children who are victims of mistreatment and ghost children. There is then a strong risk that it will be exploited by a murderous ideology. Our experience of the genocides of the 20th century has not enabled us to impede those we are witnessing currently.

Each part of reality has ascendants and descendants. The attention and respect that we show to the part of reality of our time and to its origins, our listening to its future potentialities, and the wish to understand its present, constitute factors of both anchorage and growth of the multiple aspects of this part of reality.

For the reality that we call "true" – associating with it the concept of "truth" – has infinite facets, more numerous even than those of the finite world of the neo-reality of the Bubble. But these facets obey the constraint of the time of true creation, not of imitation.

Thus, the average time of gestation of the human foetus retains its creative autonomy, whether its container is a biological mother, a surrogate mother, or an artificial uterus.

Thus, equally, and on the contrary, epigenesis is modified over three generations by traumas, and especially when they have been experienced in the pre-verbal period, but this modification is reversible by various therapeutic measures (Giacobino, 2018).

The investigation of reality is strewn with many more pitfalls than research in neo-reality. Its results are variable, often random, always unexpected, and vehicles of new enigmas. Outside our discipline, the best example of this randomness is given by research in the domain of quantum physics, where the trajectory of a particle can never be predicted.

In order to tackle this exploration of reality, a love for the living world, wonder at knowledge, and an insatiable curiosity for uncovering fragments of truth are necessary.

Love plays a primordial role in sustaining every hypothesis and idea that we believe to be new, while hate sterilizes creativity, even at the level of concrete reality: there is no greater hate than the sterilizing rape of women martyrized by outlaws who seek to make today's world the sterile soil of tomorrow, inherited by an anonymous descendance without history.

Life and death of psychoanalysis

To paraphrase the title of the book by Jean Laplanche (2001), I do not know if psychoanalysis, especially child and adolescent psychoanalysis, will still be alive a few years from now. This part of reality has occupied a major place in my investments and in my lifetime, but I must consider the possibility of being at the sickbed of a reality that is condemned to disappear. And yet, would any parent throw up their hands and stop caring for their child if they were told that the child was going to die one day – in ten days, ten years or ninety years?

The paradox of the finiteness of life resides in the possibility of touching the infinite and the eternal. Yet what is more infinite than the pressure of the drive, and more eternal than the need for relationships?

One thing is certain, the future of the reality of psychoanalysis, for all ages, is entering a new phase.

Even if he had hoped for greater successes, Freud always considered psychoanalysis as one form of psychotherapy among others and, at the level of science, as a confidential discipline. The reason for this point of view lay more in his knowledge than in modesty, real or false. The hard road that led him to his discoveries made him experience in his flesh how natural it is for the human being to repress, and even expel the experience of the supremacy of the unconscious over consciousness. I have often asked myself how he would have appreciated the immense media success that our profession enjoyed in the second half of the 20th century. If we cast an eye back today to examine the path travelled, we can better evaluate the ups and downs of this popularity.

There is no question that psychoanalytic practice has helped several generations to interest themselves in psychic life. It has also greatly contributed to reforming the old psychiatric institutions and creating new formulas of treatment, including in the domain of childhood and adolescence. Unfortunately, caught in the dazzle of the lifting of repression, we thought that the game was won, but we underestimated the colossal power of the mechanisms of defence and of the negativity of the human being.

Out of complacency with those who refused to recognize the therapeutic dimension that was so essential for Freud, we have contributed to sowing doubt about the analytic method and giving ground to more "concrete" therapies, old techniques in new clothing. By forgetting that research consists in humility and constantly calling things into question, we have contributed to the advent of ready-made formulas instead of the perpetual questioning that helped Freud to make progress in his immense work. By forgetting that the perverse tendencies of our own Infantile do not remain in the cloakroom during our professional activity, we have given them free rein rather than analysing their interaction with the Infantile in our patient of all ages.

We have thus confined ourselves within a mentality of omniscient narcissism, accompanied by a phobic avoidance of the Infantile and, in particular, infantile sexuality. This mentality characteristic of a period of latency which we are a bit old for has emptied psychoanalysis of its substance, reducing it to a subject of living-room conversation between acculturated adults. We then became the target of hateful attacks and, what is worse, our self-satisfaction was taken advantage of in order to take back one after the other each of the places that we had conquered in the domain of mental health. The unconscious saw itself reduced to a reservoir of energy, while consciousness was deflected from its aim – which is to better understand psychic functioning – and put in the service of voluntary and illusory efforts to consciously change behavior.

The absence of an overview of the measures undertaken to bring about these changes means that the "behaviourized" subject finds himself too often in the situation of the character of Fernand Raynaud in his sketch about the tailor.[2]

The suffering of children in the world today

But what is happening meanwhile in the world of children?

Four years as president of the Committee of the International Psychoanalytical Association for the Psychoanalysis of Children and Adolescents (COCAP) have enabled me to note two facts:

1 The future of the practice of psychoanalysis in general is in great danger on all the continents.

2 If we want to try and save this practice, it is through our practice with children and adolescents that we will achieve it.

In all countries, children are born; each year, malnutrition kills 3.1 million children under the age of 5; one out of four children in the world suffers from retarded growth; in the so-called developing world, 66 million children of school age go there on an empty stomach.

300,000 children in more than 40 countries are child soldiers who are used to kill and satisfy the sexual needs of adult combatants. A number of colleagues on other continents have followed up these children after their "demobilization" and have published accounts of treatments. The least that can be said about them is that their submission to the barbaric methods of their enrolment has left these children with what Marty (1991) calls an "operational" or "matter-of-fact" (*opératoire*) mode of intellectual functioning and a massive inhibition of their emotional world, in particular a pathological insensibility to suffering, both their own and that of others.

If we want psychoanalysis to live, we must listen to the children of today, relate to them and help them recognize their psychic suffering as an opportunity to develop their human relations, their knowledge and their creativity. Our training allows us to be the witnesses of a psychic reality denied by the quantitative world in which they are growing up. We can speak to them about the quality and the value of the feelings that animate them, tell them that ignorance is not a defect, any more than uncertainty, but rather that they are intermediate states that are necessary for discovering knowledge of the world and of self-development.

We are well placed to speak to them about the human community, about the resemblance of hearts and souls under the differences of skin and culture; to help them distinguish between external unhappiness and inner anxiety, and to help them discover that sadness is neither an illness nor a malediction, but rather an emotion that is necessary for progressing along the path of the recognition of reality and of self-development.

We can help them to approach the mysteries of life, the functioning of their bodies and their fear of death, with other means than skeletons, ghosts and virtual killings to which they have been accustomed since they were very young, to the point of no longer distinguishing them from killings in the world of reality.

We are in a position to familiarize them with the mystery of the force that is pulsating in them, with the illogical contradictions and conflicts that it engenders, and to show them that this energy can be transformed and diversified infinitely if one can get beyond the level zero of its expression, which is raw excitation. We can help them rediscover the natural and precious skill that is *attention*, whose connection with the advent of meaning Bion (1970) formulated brilliantly in the title of a dazzling book *Attention and Interpretation*.

Each child has received this capacity at birth; unfortunately, it has been so mishandled by the bad management of the daily life of our society as a whole that we have reached the point of regarding its deficit as a pathology – ADHD[3] – imputable to the child, whereas it is created experimentally by the social environment.

As psychoanalysts, we can give children and adolescents the chance to experience the unique quality of a personal relationship in comparison with the "millions of friends" they have on the web and, if they feel awkward in the realm of emotions, we can tell them that even this awkwardness is precious because it is a sign of the sensibility of those who feel it. We can also lead them to tell the difference between a simple performance and a true creation, between a conglomerate of bizarre objects and a work of art.

I will end my enumeration there and can already hear some people saying:

"All that is very well, but you are speaking about a parental role! And where is psychoanalysis in all that?"

At the risk of not only making friends, my answer is that psychoanalysis is very much there. Because, if we know how to go about it, children are still capable of listening and playing in other ways than simply with their game console or the mobile of their parents, of drawing their fantasies, of laughing and crying spontaneously, of getting angry and of asking for a cuddle, of getting excited and of "[sleeping], perchance to dream" (*Hamlet*, Shakespeare, Act 3, Sc. 1, 10).

Because they do not know yet how to "manage their emotions" within a perspective of erasure of the singular, because repression has not yet crushed their ego, their drives and their emotions, because they are still capable of asking about the "why" of things, it is still possible to offer their psychical life other paths of expression, of relating in another way to them, of helping them to hear another music of life than that to which they are being conditioned.

There is nothing to prevent us, of course, from speaking in the same way to the Infantile in our adult patients; it is even strongly recommended, but there our task is more difficult because we are working against the society of which they are part, in social roles that children do not have as yet.

The urgency of transformation

Now that the "thirty glorious years" of psychoanalysis are no more than a memory, we must return to the status of confidentiality that Freud had assigned to psychoanalysis.

It is up to us to transform this disenchantment of society for our discipline into an opportunity to develop ourselves, in particular, in the domain of listening to what is infraverbal, infrasymbolic, to the "memories in feelings" dear to Melanie Klein (1948), to everything that mobilizes the "normal illness" of the mother dear to Winnicott (1958).

Throughout my professional life, I have worked on the relationship between the Infantile in my patients and my own Infantile, and not only my adult parts. Indeed, it is my Infantile that suffers the instinctual drive pressure linked to my relationship with each patient, as well as to the attacks of repression, denial and splitting. It is my Infantile that experiences my movements of identification and projection in the day-to-day relationship with each of my patients. It is due to my Infantile that, owing to these movements, I find myself in blind spots of countertransference from which I must subsequently emerge, once I have learnt from them their significance and usefulness for the continuation of the analytic process. And my situation is identical to that of all psychoanalysts in all countries of the world.

Having travelled the world quite extensively, I have seen the fortunes and misfortunes of psychoanalysis in our contemporary society. It was in doing so that I acquired the conviction that, if we succeed in keeping alive a discipline that is so indispensable to the mental health of our contemporaries and our descendants, it can only be thanks to child and adolescent psychoanalysis. Getting down on the floor and on to all fours to play games with children, whose significance it will sometimes take us a long time to grasp, is well worth the trouble. It is worthwhile tolerating the small share of the cake that is accorded to us in our institutions.

Because, in this way, we will be on the side of hope and the future, it is worth accepting to be, for a further an indeterminate period . . .

. . . *nightwatchmen, for the love of the living world.*

Notes

* A first version of this text was presented in 2014 in Paris on the occasion of the twentieth anniversary of the European Psychoanalytic Society for Children and Adolescents (SEPEA), and published in the volume of commemoration of this event: *Psychanalyse de l'enfant et de l'adolescent. Psychanalyse de l'enfant et de l'adolescent. État des lieux et perspectives* (Guignard, 2017).

1 Louis Jouvet (1887–1951) actor and stage director.

2 For those who do not know it, it concerns a man who returns to see his tailor to complain that "there "appears to be a defect" in the suit that has just been delivered to him. The tailor manages to persuade the man to contort himself more and more in order to adapt himself to his suit which, in reality is poorly cut. The punchline of the sketch is edifying: ""I'm lucky", the man exclaims, "to have found a tailor capable of dressing such a wretched fellow as I!"

3 Attention Deficit Disorder / (with or without) Hyperactivity.

Chapter 16

Conclusion

During the ordinary day of a psychoanalyst, images, words and affects appear in apparent disorder, yet organized by each transference/countertransference relationship. This relationship is homologous with the neurotic relationship that each patient has with the traumatic environment of his past. Thus, as the hours go by, the analyst walks through landscapes that are extremely varied yet similar, in the respiration and palpitation of human psychic life.

He will only be able to respond validly to the expectation that he perceives in those who have decided to work with him, for so long and with so much effort, by taking this roundabout path, the longest route, which, quite naturally, passes through childhood. Yes, but whose childhood? Logic, plain logic, requires us to answer: the patient's childhood, of course. And, certainly, that is the vital minimum of a therapeutic relationship, irrespective of the technique used.

However, I am inclined to believe now that what constitutes the specificity of the psychoanalytic technique is in the order of this encounter, contained within the analytic setting, of two Infantiles, that of the analysand and that of the analyst. The narcissistic and object-related issues at stake in this encounter are considerable and totally asymmetrical: the life of one of them will acquire substance through the struggle with, and then the abandonment of, the other. This other, the analyst, has the delicate task of transferring, discretely and without countertransference violence, to the internal objects of his analysand what the latter has confided in him unwittingly in the incessant movement of the infantile transference. He can only do so on the express condition of remaining in contact with his own Infantile. It is the latter that will enable him to guarantee his patient the whole range of questionings and sufferings related to the discovery of the differences – between the sexes and the generations – that punctuate human evolution in its solitude and uniqueness. It will be for the reader to say if the heart of this Infantile has, like quicksilver, run right through the pages of this book.

References

Abraham, K. (1924). A brief study of the development of the libido in the light of mental disorders: maniac-depressive states and pregenital levels of Libido. In: K. Abraham, E. Jones, D. Bryan, & A. Stachey (Eds.) (1949), *Selected Papers of Karl Abraham*. London: Hogarth, pp. 418–501.

Alleon, A.-M., Morvan, O. & Lebovici, S. (1990). *Devenir " adulte "?* Paris: Presses Universitaires de France.

Anzieu, D. (1994). *Le Penser. Du Moi-peau au Moi-pensant*. Paris: Dunod, 2013.

Arnoux, D. & Jean, C. (1985). Corps souffrant. *Adolescence*, 4: 267–283.

Barande, I. (1977). *Le Maternel singulier*. Paris: Aubier-Montaigne.

Barande, R. (1989). *Parcours d'un psychanalyste*. Paris: Pro-Edi.

Baranes, J.-J. (1993). Deveni soi-même: avatars et statut du transgénérationnel. In: R. Kaës (Ed.), *Transmission de la vie psychique entre les générations*. Paris: Dunod, pp. 70–190.

Baranger, M. & Baranger, W. (2008). The analytic situation as a dynamic field 1961–62. *International Journal of Psychoanalysis*, 89(4): 795–826.

Begoin, J. (1982). L'interprétation de la réalité psychique. *Revue française de psychanalyse*, 46(5): 1003–1022.

Begoin-Guignard, F. (1981). Pulsions sadiques et pulsions épistémophiliques. In: H. Sztulman (Ed.), *La Curiosité en psychanalyse*. Toulouse: Privat.

Begoin-Guignard, F. (1987). À l'aube du maternel et du féminin. Essai sur deux concepts aussi évidents qu'inconcevables. *Revue française de psychanalyse*, 51(6): 1491–1503.

Bellay, J. du (1558). *Les Regrets, 1553–1557*. Paris: Morel.

Bentinck van Schoonheten, A. (2018). *Karl Abraham: Life and Work, A Biography*, trans. Liz Walters. London: Routledge.

Bergeret, J. (1976). Dépressivité et dépression dans le cadre de l'économie défensive. *Revue française de psychanalyse*, 40(5–6): 835–1044.

Bernateau, I. (2017). *Lieux, non-lieux et anti-lieux à l'adolescence*. Week-end SEPEA 2017 Enreg. Congrès-minute, congresminute.com

Bion, W.R. (1961). *Experiences in Groups*. London: Tavistock.

Bion, W.R. (1962a). *Learning from Experience*. London: Heinemann.

Bion, W.R. (1962b). A theory of thinking. *International Journal of Psychoanalysis*, 43: 306–310. Reprinted in: Bion: 1967, pp. 110–119.

Bion, W.R. (1963). *Elements of Psycho-Analysis*. London: Heinemann.

Bion, W.R. (1965). *Transformations. Change from Learning to Growth*. London: Heinemann.
Bion, W.R. (1967). *Second Thoughts: Selected Papers on Psycho-Analysis*. London: Heinemann.
Bion, W.R. (1970). *Attention and Interpretation*. London: Tavistock.
Bion, W.R. (1992). *Cogitations*. London: Karnac.
Bion, W.R. (2005). *The Tavistock Seminars, 1976–1979*. London: Karnac.
Bléandonu, G. et al. (1992). *Cadres thérapeutiques et enveloppes psychiques: quatrièmes journées d'étude francophones sur les hôpitaux de jour*. Lyon: Pu de Lyon.
Bokanowski, Th. (1995). Le couple "trauma-clivage" in the *Journal clinique de Ferenczi*. In: T. Bokanowski, K. Kelley-Laîné, et al. (Eds.), *Sándor Ferenczi*, Monographies de la Revue française de psychanalyse. Paris: Presses Universitaires de France.
Bokanowski, Th. (1996). Théories de l'enfant, enfants de la théorie. *Études freudiennes*, 37: 151–163.
Braunschweig, D. & Fain, M. (1971). *Éros et Ánteros. Réflexions psychanalytiques sur la sexualité*. Paris: Payot.
Braunschweig, D. & Fain, M. (1975). *La Nuit, le Jour*. Paris: Presses Universitaires de France.
Brusset, B. (1992). *Le Développement libidinal*. Paris: Presses Universitaires de France.
Brusset, B. (1994). L'enfant, l'infantile et la causalité psychique. *Revue française de psychanalyse*, 58(3): 693–705.
Cahn, R. (1991). *Adolescence et folie*. Paris: Presses Universitaires de France.
Carroll, L. (1869). *Alice's Adventures in Wonderland*. Boston: Lee Shepard.
Chasseguet-Smirgel, J. (1967). *Pour une psychanalyse de l'art et de la créativité*. Paris: Payot.
Clarapède, E. (1905). *Le Jeu chez l'Enfant*. Neuchâtel and Paris: Delachaux & Niestlé.
Denis, P. (2002). *Emprise et satisfaction. Les deux formants de la pulsion*. Paris: Presses Universitaires de France.
Diatkine, R. & Simon, J. (1972). *La Psychanalyse précoce*. Paris: Presses Universitaires de France.
Donnet, J.-L. (1995). *Le Divan bien tempéré*. Paris: Presses Universitaires de France.
Donnet, J.-L. (2005). *La Situation analysante*. Paris: Presses Universitaires de France.
Echenoz, J. (1979). *Le méridien de Greenwich*. Paris: Minuit.
Ehrensaft, D. (2014). Family complexes and oedipal circles: mothers, fathers, babies, donors, and surrogates. In: M. Mann et al. (Eds.), *Psychoanalytic Aspects of Assisted Reproductive Technology*. London: Karnac.
Fairbairn, W.R.D. (1952). *Psychoanalytic Studies of the Personality*. London: Routledge.
Feldman, M. (2009). *Doubt, Conviction and the Analytic Process*. London: Routledge.
Ferro, A. (1996). *La Psychanalyse comme oeuvre ouverte. Emotions, récits, transformations*. Ramonville: Erès, 2000.
Forman, M.B. (Ed.). (1952). *The Letters of John Keats*. London: Oxford University Press.
Freud, S. (1895) (with Breuer). *Studies in Hysteria*. *S.E.* 2. London: Hogarth.
Freud, S. (1900). *The Interpretation of Dreams*. *S.E.* 4 and 5. London: Hogarth, pp. 1–621.

Freud, S. (1905). *Three Essays on the Theory of Sexuality. S.E.* 7. London: Hogarth, pp. 130–243.
Freud, S. (1909). *Analysis of a Phobia in a Five-year-old Boy. S.E. 10.* London: Hogarth, pp. 5–149.
Freud, S. (1910). *Leonardo da Vinci and a Memory of his Childhood. SE.* 11. London: Hogarth, pp. 57–137.
Freud, S. (1911). *Formulations on the Two Principles of Mental Functioning. S.E.* 12. London: Hogarth, pp. 218–226.
Freud, S. (1912). *A Note on the Unconscious in Psychoanalysis. S.E.* 12. London: Hogarth, pp. 255–257.
Freud, S. (1914). *Remembering, Repeating, Working-through. S.E.* 12. London: Hogarth, pp. 145–156.
Freud, S. (1915a). *Instincts and their Vicissitudes. S.E.* 14. London: Hogarth, pp. 109–140.
Freud, S. (1915b). *Repression. S.E.* 14. London: Hogarth, pp. 141–158.
Freud, S. (1915c). *The unconscious. S.E.* 14. London: Hogarth, pp. 166–215.
Freud, S. (1917a [1915]). *Mourning and Melancholia. S.E.* 14. London: Hogarth, pp. 237–260.
Freud, S. (1917b [1915]). *A Metapsychological Supplement to the Theory of Dreams.* S.E. 14, pp. 222–235.
Freud, S. (1918 [1914]). *From the History of an Infantile Neurosis. S.E.* 17. London: Hogarth, pp. 7–122.
Freud, S. (1919). *'The "Uncanny"'. S.E.* 17. London: Hogarth, pp. 217–252.
Freud, S. (1920). *Beyond the Pleasure Principle. S.E.* 18. London: Hogarth, pp. 1–64.
Freud, S. (1921). *Group Psychology and the Analysis of the Ego. S.E.* 18. London: Hogarth, pp. 65–143.
Freud, S. (1923a). *The Ego and the Id. S.E.* 19. London: Hogarth, pp. 1–66.
Freud, S. (1923b). *The Infantile Genital Organization. S.E.* 19. London: Hogarth, pp. 141–145.
Freud, S. (1924). *The Economic Problem of Masochism. S.E.* 19. London: Hogarth, pp. 155–170.
Freud, S. (1926a [1925]). *Psycho-Analysis (An Article in the Encyclopaedia Britannica). S.E. 20.* London: Hogarth, pp. 263–270.
Freud, S. (1926b [1925]). *Inhibitions, Symptoms and Anxiety. S.E.* 20. London: Hogarth, pp. 75–174.
Freud, S. (1937). *Analysis Terminable and Interminable. S.E.* 23. London: Hogarth, pp. 209–253.
Freud, S. (1940 [1938]). *The Splitting of the Ego in the Process of Defence'. S.E.* 23. London: Hogarth, pp. 271–278.
Freud, S. (1950 [1895]). *Project for a Scientific Psychology. S.E.* 1. London: Hogarth, pp. 281–397.
Gammill, J. (2007). *La Position dépressive au service de la vie.* Paris: In Press.
Giacobino, A. (2018). *Peut-on se libérer de ses gènes? L'épigénétique.* Paris: Stock.
Gibeault, A. (1989). Destins de la symbolisation. *Revue française de psychanalyse,* 53(6): 1493–1617.
Gillibert, J. (1977). De l'auto-érotisme. *Revue française de psychanalyse,* 41(5/6): 773–949.
Girard, J.-Y. (1995). *La Machine de Turing.* Paris: Seuil.

Green, A. (1973 [1999]). *The Fabric of Affect in the Psychoanalytic Discourse*, trans. A. Sheridan. London: Routledge.

Green, A. (1983). *Life Narcissism, Death Narcissism*, trans. A. Weller. London: Free Association Books, 2001.

Green, A. (1988). Pulsions, psyché, langage, pensée. *Revue française de psychanalyse*, 52(2): 491–497.

Green, A. (1993). *The Work of the Negative*, trans. A. Weller. London: Free Association Books.

Green, J. (1949). *If I Were You*, trans. J.H.F. McEwen. New York: Harper & Bros.

Grinberg, L. (1962). On a specific aspect of countertransference due to the patient's projective identification. *International Journal of Psychoanalysis*, 43: 436–440.

Grinberg, L. (2018). *Qui a peur du contre-transfert?* Paris: Ithaque.

Grotstein, J. (2007). *A Beam of Intense Darkness. Wilfred Bion's Legacy to Psychoanalysis*. London: Karnac.

Grunberger, B. (1971). *Le Narcissisme*. Paris: Payot.

Grunberger, B. (1989). *Narcisse et Anubis*. Paris: Éditions des Femmes.

Guignard, F. (1972). Les troubles de la signification chez les débiles mentaux (II), *Revue française de psychanalyse*, 36(5–6): 879–881.

Guignard, F. (1985). Ballade au Préconscient. *Revue française de psychanalyse*, (5): 1391–1400.

Guignard, F. (1986). Le Sourire du chat. Réflexions sur le féminin à partir de la pratique analytique quptidienne. In: Guignard, 1997a, Épître à l'objet, Paris, Presses Universitaires de France pp. 129–145.

Guignard, F. (1988). Le rôle des identifications maternelles et féminines dans le devenir du masculin chez le garçon. *Adolescence*, 6(1): 49–74.

Guignard, F. (1989). Enjeux de la symbolisation à l'adolescence. *Revue française de psychanalyse*, 53(6): 1755–1761.

Guignard, F. (1994a). Les pièges de la représentation dans l'interprétation psychanalytique. *Journal psychanalytique de l'enfant*, 15: 139–153.

Guignard, F. (1994b). L'enfant dans le psychanalyste. *Revue française de psychanalyse*, 58(3): 649–659.

Guignard, F. (1995a). The Infantile in the analytic relationship. *International Journal of Psycho-Analysis*, 76: 1083–1093.

Guignard, F. (1995b). Prégénitalité et scène primitive, ou le destin fantasmatique du *tractus* digestif. *Revue française de psychanalyse*, 59(3): 771–784; reprinted in Guignard, 1996a.

Guignard, F. (1996). *Au vif de l'Infantile*. Paris: Delachaux et Niestlé.

Guignard, F. (1997a). *Épître à l'objet*. Paris: Presses Universitaires de France.

Guignard, F. (1997b). Adolescence de la féminité. In: *Guignard*, 1997a, pp. 11–128.

Guignard, F. (2002). La magie des gros mots. *Revue Humoresques, Santé du Rire*, 16: 29–37.

Guignard, F. (2015). A commentary on Giuseppe Givitarese's paper, "Transformations in hallucinosis and the receptivity of the analyst". *International Journal of Psychoanalysis*, 96(4): 1117–1124.

Guignard, F. (2017). Psychanalyse de l'enfant et de l'adolescent. In: *Psychanalyse de l'enfant et de l'adolescent. État des lieux et perspectives*. Paris: In Press, 2017.

Guignard, F. (2020). *Psychoanalytic Concepts and Technique in Development: Psychoanalysis, Neuroscience and Physics*, trans. A. Weller. London: Routledge.

Guignard, F., De Ajurliaguerra, J., Jaeggi, A., Kocher, F., Maquard, M., Roth, S. & Sschmid- Kitsikis, E. (1965). Évolution et pronostic de la dysphasie chez l'enfant. *La Psychiatrie de l'Enfant*, 8(2): 391–452.

Guignard, F., Garrone, G., Haeberli, A.–M., Perrin, C. & Rodriguez, R., (1972). Les troubles de la signification chez les débiles mentaux (I). *La Psychiatrie de l'Enfant*, 14(1): 879–881.

Gutton, P. (1991). *Le Pubertaire*. Paris: Presses Universitaires de France.

Haag, G. (2018). *Le Moi corporel: à partir de la clinique de l'autisme et de l'observation du premier développement*. Paris: Presses Universitaires de France.

Jones, E. (1953–1957). *The Life and Work of Sigmund Freud*, Vols. 1–3. New York: Basic Book.

Jouvet, M. (1992). *Le Sommeil et le rêve*. Paris: Odile Jacob, 2000.

Kestemberg, E. & Kestemberg, J. (1966). Contribution à la perspective génétique en psychanalyse. *Revue française de psychanalyse*, 30(5–6): 569–574.

Kestemberg, E., Kestemberg, J. & Decobert, S. (1972). *La Faim et le corps*. Paris: Presses Universitaires de France.

King, P. & Steiner, R. (1991). *The Freud-Klein Controversies, 1941–1945*. London: Routledge.

Klein, M. (1921). The development of a child. In: Klein, 1975, pp. 1–53.

Klein, M. (1923). Early analysis. In: Klein, 1975, pp. 77–105.

Klein, M. (1926). The psychological principles of early analysis. In: Klein, 1975, pp. 128–138.

Klein, M. (1928). Early stages of the Oedipus conflict. In: Klein, 1975, pp. 186–198.

Klein, M. (1929). Personification in the play of children. In: Klein, 1975, pp. 199–209.

Klein, M. (1930). The importance of symbol-formation in the development of the ego. In: Klein, 1975, pp. 219–232.

Klein, M. (1931). A contribution to the theory of intellectual inhibition. In: Klein, 1975, pp. 236–247.

Klein, M. (1932). *The Psychoanalysis of Children*, trans. A. Strachey. London: Hogarth Press and the Institute of Psycho-Analysis, 1986.

Klein, M. (1933). The early development of conscience in the child. In: Klein, 1975, pp. 248–257.

Klein, M. (1940). Mourning and its relation to manic-depressive states. In: Klein, 1975, pp. 344–369.

Klein, M. (1945). The Oedipus complex in the light of early anxieties. In: Klein, 1975, pp. 370–419.

Klein, M. (1946). Notes on some schizoid mechanisms. In: *Envy and Gratitude and Other Papers, 1946–1963. The Writings of Melanie Klein*, Vol. III. London: Hogarth, pp. 1–25.

Klein, M. (1948). On the theory of anxiety and guilt. In: Klein, Heimann et al. (Eds.), 1952, pp. 271–291.

Klein, M. (1952). Some theoretical conclusions regarding the emotional life of the infant. In: Klein, 1957, pp. 61–94.

Klein, M. (1957). *Envy and Gratitude and Other Papers, 1921–45. The Writings of Melanie Klein*, Vol. III. London: Hogarth.

Klein, M. (1975). *Love, Guilt and Reparation and other works, 1921–1945*. London: Hogarth.

Klein, M. & Heimann, P. (1952). *Developments in Psychoanalysis*. London: Hogarth.

Kreisler, L., Fain, M. & Soule, M. (1966). La clinique psychosomatique de l'enfant. À propos des troubles fonctionnels du nourrisson. *Psychiatrie de l'enfant*, 9(1): 89–222.

Kundera, M. (1984). *L'Insoutenable légèreté de l'être*. Paris: Gallimard.

Lacan, J. (1966). *Écrits*, trans. B. Fink. New York: Norton & Co., 2002.

Lacan, J. (1969). *Séminaire XVI: D'un à l'Autre*. Paris: Seuil.

Ladame, F. & Jeammet, P. (1986). *La Psychiatrie de l'adolescence aujourd'hui. Quels adolescents soigner et comment?* Paris: Presses Universitaires de France.

Lamartine de, A. (1817). Le Lac. *Œuvres poétiques complètes*. Paris: Gallimard, Bibliothèque de la Pléiade, 1963 (English quotation source: http://feherilles.blogspot.hu).Laplanche, J. (1981). *Problématiques IV: L'Inconscient et le ça*. Paris: Presses Universitaires de France, 1998.

Laplanche, J. (2001). *Vie et mort en psychanalyse*. Paris: Flammarion.

Laplanche, J. & Pontalis, J.-B. (1967). *The Language of Psychoanalysis*. London: Hogarth, 1973.

Laufer, M. & Laufer, M.E. (1989). *Adolescence et rupture du développement. Une perspective psychanalytique*. Paris: Presses Universitaires de France.

Mancia, M. (2007). Mémoire implicite et inconscient précoce non refoulé: leur rôle dans le transfert et le rêve. *Revue française de psychanalyse*, 71(2): 369–388.

Marty, P. (1991). *Mentalisation et psychosomatique*. Paris: Les Empêcheurs de penser en rond.

Masson, J.M. (Ed.). (1985). *The Complete Letters of Sigmund Freud to Wilhelm Fliess, 1887–1904*. Cambridge, MA: Belknap.

Matte Blanco, I. (1975). *The Unconscious as Infinite Sets. An Essay in Bi-logic*. Londres: Duckworth.

Meltzer, D. (1967). *The Psychoanalytic Process*. London: Karnac.

Meltzer, D. (1973). *Sexual States of Mind*. London: Karnac, 2008.

Meltzer, D. (1978). The clinical significance of the work of Bion. In: D. Meltzer (Ed.) (1972–1978), *The Kleinian Development of Psychoanalysis*, Part 3. London: Karnac, 1998.

Meltzer, D. (1983). *Studies in Extended Metapsychology*. Perthshire: Clunie Press.

Meltzer, D. (1992). *The Claustrum. An Investigation of Claustrophobic Phenomena*. With an Essay by Meg Harris Williams: Shakespeare's Equivocation, Macbeth's Ambiguity. London: Karnac, 2008.

Meltzer, D. & Williams, M.H. (1988). *The Apprehension of Beauty: The Role of Aesthetic Conflict in Art, Development and Violence*. London: Karnac.

Money-Kyrle, (1956). Normal concepts of counter-transference and some of its deviations. *International Journal of Psychoanalysis*, 37(4–5): 360–366.

Neyraut, M. (1978). *Les logiques de l'inconscient*. Paris: Hachette.

Ogden, Th. (1994). *Subjects of Analysis*. London: Karnac.

Ogden, Th. (1997). *Reverie and Interpretation: Sensing Something Human*. Northvale, NJ: Jason Aronson/Londres: Karnac.

Ogden, Th. (2004). The analytic third: implications for psychoanalytic theory and technique. *Psychoanalytic Quarterly*, 73(1): 167–195.

Ortoli, S. & Pharabod, J.-P. (1984). *La Cantique des Quantiques*. Paris: La Découverte.

Parat, C. (1987). À propos de la co-excitation libidinale. *Revue française de psychanalyse*, 51(3): 925–935.

Piaget, J. (1950). *La Construction du réel chez l'enfant*. Neuchâtel and Paris: Delachaux & Niestlé.

Pontalis, J. (1998). *L'Enfant des limbes*. Paris: Gallimard.

Rimbaud, A. (1871). Lettre du voyant. In: *Œuvres complètes*. Paris: Gallimard, Bibliothèque de la Pléiade.

Rosenfeld, H. (1965). *Psychotic States*. London: Karnac.

Rosenfeld, H. (1987). *Impasse and Interpretation. Therapeutic and Anti-therapeutic Factors in the Psychoanalytic Treatment of Psychotic, Borderline and Neurotic Patients*. London: Tavistock.

Schmid-Kitsikis, E. (1995). Des hommes et des pères... À propos du rôle déflecteur de l'objet. *Revue française de psychanalyse*, 59, spécial Congrès.

Segal, H. (1957) Notes on symbol formation, *Int. J. Psycho-Anal.*, 38, 391–397.

Segal, H. (1990). *Dream, Phantasy and Art*. London: Routledge.

Spitz, R. (1965). *The First Year of Life. A Psychoanalytic Study of Normal and Deviant Development in Object Relations*. New York: International Universities Press.

Tisseron, S. (2001). *L'Intimité surexposée*. Paris: Ramsay.

Tisseron, S. (2012). *Rêver, fantasmer, virtualiser, du virtuel psychique au virtuel numérique*. Paris: Dunod.

Troisier, H. (1991). Entretien avec Jean Favreau. *Revue française de psychanalyse*, 54(1): 189–196.

Verlazza, N. (Ed.). (2019). *Paul Verlaine: A Bilingual Selection of his Verse*, trans. S.N. Rosenberg. Pennsylvania: The Pennsylvania State University Press.

Viderman, S. (1970). *La Construction de l'espace analytique*. Paris: Denoël.

Vinci, L. da (c. 1490–1519). *Trattaro della Pittura, Vatican Library*. See Ludwig, H. (1909).

Vinci, L. da (1651) *Traité de la peinture*, éd. d'Anna Sconza, Paris, Les Belles Lettres, coll. « Le cabinet des images », 2012, 464 p.

Widlöcher, D. (2013). Empathie et co-pensée. *Journal de la psychanalyse de l'enfant*, 3(2): 39–44.

Winnicott, D.W. (1958). *Through Paediatrics to Psychoanalysis: Collected Papers*. London: Tavistock.

Winnicott, D.W. (1960). Ego-distortion in terms of true and false self. In: Winnicott, 1965, pp. 140–152.

Winnicott, D.W. (1965). *The Maturational Processes and the Facilitating Environment*. London: Karnac, 1990.

Index